'should be required reading for students of how we've managed to get it all so horribly wrong'
Sunday Business Post

'rewarding reading'
Zoo

'an absorbing read'
www.ShortList.com

'No one who reads this book will feel untouched by its findings, and with any luck, will change their lives before it's too late'
www.theresident.co.uk

'an absorbing and effective wake-up call'
London Lite

'entertaining reading'
London Paper

'compelling'
Psychologies

'fascinating food for thought'
First

Praise for *The Selfish Capitalist*

'many of us will have a great deal of sympathy with what James is trying to tell us'
Daily Mail

'our foremost chronicler of what ails us'
Will Self

'His most serious work . . . the message is that goaded by advertising we constantly confuse wants with needs. We should do things because they give us pleasure, he believes, not because they promise the empty prizes of possessions or status'
The Times

Also by Oliver James:

Juvenile Violence in a Winner–Loser Culture
Britain on the Couch
They F*** You Up
Affluenza
The Selfish Capitalist

For further information about Oliver James and his work see:
www.oliver-james-books.com

Contented Dementia

Oliver James

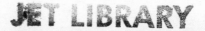

Vermilion
LONDON

9 10 8

First published in 2008 by Vermilion, an imprint of Ebury Publishing
This edition published by Vermilion in 2009

Ebury Publishing is a Random House Group company

The Random House Group Limited Reg. No. 954009

Addresses for companies within the Random House Group can be found at www.randomhouse.co.uk

A CIP catalogue record for this book is available from the British Library

The Random House Group Limited supports the Forest Stewardship Council® (FSC®), the leading international forest certification organisation. All our titles that are printed on Greenpeace approved FSC® certified paper carry the FSC® logo. Our paper procurement policy can be found at www.randomhouse.co.uk/environment

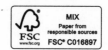

Printed in the UK by CPI Mackays, Chatham, ME5 8TD

ISBN 9780091901813

Copies are available at special rates for bulk orders. Contact the sales development team on 020 7840 8487 for more information.

To buy books by your favourite authors and register for offers, visit www.randomhouse.co.uk

The information in this book has been compiled by way of general guidance in relation to the specific subjects addressed, but is not a substitute and not to be relied on for medical, healthcare, pharmaceutical or other professional advice on specific circumstances and in specific locations. Please consult your GP before changing, stopping or starting any medical treatment. So far as the author is aware the information given is correct and up to date as at June 2008. Practice, laws and regulations all change, and the reader should obtain up to date professional advice on any such issues. The author and publishers disclaim, as far as the law allows, any liability arising directly or indirectly from the use, or misuse, of the information contained in this book.

This is a work of non-fiction. The names of people in the case studies have been changed solely to protect the privacy of others.

To Dorothy

An Open Letter from Penelope Garner, Inventor of the Method Described in this Book, for Readers who have been Diagnosed as Having Dementia

Dear Reader,

If you have been diagnosed with dementia and have picked up this book, this is a letter specially for you.

You are the expert in a most extraordinary subject – dementia. Your memory is behaving quite strangely and letting you down. You know what it's like to be slightly out of step in a way that is sometimes difficult to describe.

This book is designed for other people to learn what you already know, so that they can help rather than hinder your progress through life.

Here, below, are a few tips specially for you. Stick to these, and you can safely leave everything else in the hands of the person you trust most.

1. **From now on please don't worry about the future** – stay with what you already know and love.
2. **Appoint the person you most trust as your advocate** – and ask them to read this book while you get on with your life.
3. **Forget all about the diagnosis** – you're very good at forgetting now, so use this skill to forget about dementia and get on with enjoying your life once more.

If you take these tips to heart you have nothing to fear. Be confident, go with the flow and leave all the work to someone else.

With Very Best Wishes,
Penelope Garner

CONTENTS

Introduction

The idea of dementia sends a chill down the spine, like no other ailment.

Media coverage is uniformly pessimistic. Dramas and documentaries on television depict a gradual disintegration into non-existence; the press chronicles horror stories. Alas, this only reflects the reality of most sufferers and their carers. As the first slips of short-term memory begin to be undeniable and unmistakable, an emotional Hades beckons, because at present there is no cure and the conventional management of the illness holds out no hope of well-being. When Terry Pratchett, Britain's bestselling fiction writer, recently gave a press conference to announce he is in the early stages of the illness at the young age of 59, he said he envied his father's death through cancer. To him, Alzheimer's was 'like stripping away your living self a bit at a time . . . a nasty disease, surrounded by shadows and small, largely unseen tragedies'.

Until I met my mother-in-law, Penny Garner, I would have assumed the same. Today, I know that the disability created by dementia does not have to be hellish, that it truly is possible to create well-being for the rest of the person's life, if you use her method for managing it.

Penny was a Cotswold housewife without a university degree when she got started, nearly twenty years ago. The inspiration was the dementia of her mother, Dorothy. This single case taught her all the fundamental skills she needed. She went on to develop them working with older people at the community hospital in Burford, Oxfordshire, initially as an Alzheimer's Society helper. Through painstaking observation of what helped and what distressed the patients, she put the pieces of her theory together and turned them into a unique practice. In 1997, the work of SPECAL was described by the Alzheimer's Society as 'a very impressive demonstration of person-centred care' and 'a unique service with a model emphasis on highly individualised, person-centred care'.[1] In 1999, its effectiveness was verified and commended by a Royal College of Nursing evaluation.[2] When the National Health Service sought to sell Burford Hospital in 2002, Penny persuaded a benefactor to provide the funds which enabled her charity SPECAL (Specialized Early Care for Alzheimer's) to buy the hospital site so that her work could continue. Today, SPECAL is an internationally admired centre of excellence.

Over a period of a year, I observed Penny teaching her method to carers and professionals, and I interviewed her extensively. This book is an attempt to make the SPECAL method available to anyone who cares for a person with dementia. In particular, I hope it helps their spouses, partners, offspring and siblings, some of whom will be full-time, live-in carers, others orchestrating care from a distance.

[1] John, J., and Pride, L., 1997, 'SPECAL Project Care Service Review', Care Consortium Alzheimer's Disease Society.
[2] Pritchard, E.J. and Dewing, J., 1999, 'A Multi-Method Evaluation of the SPECAL Service for People with Dementia' (RCNI Report No.19), Oxford: Royal College of Nursing Institute.

Whatever your precise role, you will probably feel foreboding, despair and exhaustion. Worst of all you may feel you have suffered a bereavement: the person you once knew does not seem to be there any more. But I hope that by the end of the book you will see that, however advanced the illness, the real person who means so much to you is still there. This is Penny's revelation: that a great deal of the mind and emotional self of the person with dementia is still functioning as well as it ever did.

PENNY'S METHOD IN A NUTSHELL

Penny's single most important point is that the only difference between the person with dementia today and the person you used to know is a single disability: *they can no longer store new information efficiently*. All their difficulties and your problems in dealing with them derive from this fact. As you will see in Chapters 4–6, if you cease requiring them to store new information when communicating with them, a great many of the problems will disappear. To do so, you merely have to obey Penny's three commandments:

1. Don't ask questions.
2. Learn from them as the experts on their disability.
3. Always agree with everything they say, never interrupting them.

This entails replacing the common sense way we normally communicate with what Penny calls SPECALSENSE.

SPECALSENSE provides a rich vein of alternatives based on her second great discovery: *memories from long ago are still there, largely undamaged and intact.* Recent scientific studies using advanced brain imaging techniques[3] have proven what Penny has been saying for 20 years: that old memories in people with dementia are often untouched by the illness. Once you grasp this fact, not only does it greatly clarify much of what the person with dementia says and does, it also provides a key with which to unlock their isolation and ill-being. As you will see in Chapters 7–9, it enables you to help them to make sense of their surroundings and to actually enjoy their life: to permanently occupy a state of contented dementia.

In plain language, people with dementia are often using past experiences to make sense of the present, and the SPECAL method makes a virtue of this. In the absence of the new information which they have not been storing, they naturally search for past situations to provide them with a context, to indicate what the hell is going on – the fundamentals that the rest of us completely take for granted, such as: Who are these people around me? Where is this place? What is it? In the absence of recently stored clues, in a roomful of people they may look to the past and conclude that they are in an airport lounge waiting for an aeroplane. If they are at a loose end at home and have always enjoyed gardening or crosswords or Bridge or golf, they may decide that this is what they were about to do, even though their carer considers them long since incapable of such activities. So long as they are appropriately supported in their perception of what is happening, they can find themselves living as happily as they ever did. But that does not mean they will be consigned to a permanent time warp. If Penny's techniques are employed, they do not lose track

---

[3] For recent scientific papers illustrating this point, see Fleischman, D. A. et al, 2005, 'Implicit Memory and Alzheimer's Disease Neuropathology', *Brain*, 128, pp. 2006–15; and Golby, A., 2005, 'Memory Encoding in Alzheimer's Disease: an fMRI Study of Explicity and Implicit Memory', *Brain*, 128, pp. 773–87.

completely of present-day reality as experienced by the rest of us. It is possible to help them to connect their historically based way of perceiving situations with the necessary tasks of everyday living, like eating, going to the loo and sleeping. In a phrase, Penny's method 'makes a present of the past'.

Eventually, in most cases, it becomes essential to move the person to a nursing home for their own benefit (explained in Part Three). This is not fatalism but realism. It does not signify the end of your relationship. On the contrary, it signals a wise investment in your loved one's future and the basis for continuing togetherness. At this stage, it is in their best interests to be with their peers, so long as they are assisted by informed carers working on a rota system. Thankfully, it is eminently feasible to transfer the SPECAL package developed at home to the nursing home, making the job of the staff much easier.

For this book is not only intended for relatives who are carers. Anyone who has regular contact with a person with dementia at any stage of the illness should benefit. There are numerous professionals who do so, from GPs to community psychiatric nurses to carers working in nursing homes. These latter should find this book especially helpful, since responding to people with dementia is one of their main daily tasks. Several hundred such professionals, together with volunteers, have already found SPECAL training of inestimable value. Professionals encountering the SPECAL method for the first time may feel that it represents an unrealistic amount of work, given their already large caseload. Yet the reality is that so much can be achieved by the family working with their one person with dementia, supported by a SPECAL-aware professional.

This is not in any way to decry the work of the millions of people around the country who support people with dementia and are unaware of the SPECAL method. All carers should access the impressive support services to be found at local level.[4] The Alzheimer's Society, Age Concern, Help the Aged and other charities provide crucial and invaluable advice on how to obtain practical support – from accessing funding for nursing help, to provision of transport, to obtaining meals on wheels. As soon as a diagnosis has been obtained, it is vital that carers make contact with these organisations and get all the logistical back-up they can. What Penny's method confers on top of this is sustainable well-being for both the person with dementia and their carer.

The management method, beginning with basic principles and extending to specific skills and techniques, will be needed by any carer who wishes to help rather than hinder a person with a progressive irreversible dementia as they struggle to make sense of their life. SPECAL offers a particular cocktail of ingredients chosen to suit the condition, and to compensate for the disability. In the relatively early stage of dementia, where there is comparatively little disability, little compensation will be required. If the cocktail is prepared early, it will be ready on tap as more is needed later on. The earlier it is introduced, the easier the fit with the routines of everyday life. In almost all cases where dementia has been diagnosed, the problems are already advancing and the SPECAL method is your best chance of nurturing lifelong well-being. It is extremely common for family members to be unaware of the extent to which the person with dementia is disabled. People with dementia get highly skilled at concealing the situation they face, whilst being only too painfully aware of its existence. The sooner that the family engages with the

[4] Policies differ across all four countries within the UK and compared with the Republic of Ireland in regards to statutory benefits and the assessment and funding of continuing or long-term care, so I have kept mention of specific policies to a minimum.

SPECAL method, the better it will be in terms of the quality of life for all concerned, and the greater the likelihood of sustaining well-being through the rest of the person's life.

WHAT IS DEMENTIA?

The commonest dementia, known as Alzheimer's, affects 4 per cent of all retired people and a fifth of over-85s – about 700,000 Britons. The word dementia derives from the Latin words *dis*, meaning 'away from', and *mens*, meaning 'mind'. First used in the 18th century, it referred to mental deterioration and idiocy caused by the death of brain tissues. In practice, dementia is really just a word for depleted mental functioning, like memory loss or short attention span, particularly common in the elderly. While it can have several causes, such as burst blood vessels (i.e., strokes) it was not until the beginning of the twentieth century that a German neurologist, Alois Alzheimer, discovered the specific brain damage that now bears his name. Conducting an autopsy, he identified a particular pattern of neuronal tangling and degeneration.

The deficits in psychological functioning that are deemed symptoms of dementia are commonly listed as: memory loss, short attention span, disorientation, impaired judgement, illogical thinking, incapacity for abstract thought, emotional responses that seem inappropriate and incapacity to perform the activities of everyday life. All of these are associated with ageing generally, but in Alzheimer's and other dementias the decline in functioning is much more rapid.

Whereas people who have suffered strokes can recover, some-times completely, there is no cure for Alzheimer's, nor any sign of one.

At best, the drugs that have been developed to reduce the symptoms work only for a limited number of sufferers, and then just briefly. Management of the disease is already a huge problem for everyone concerned – sufferers, relatives, the health and social services – and it is set to become an ever-greater one as the elderly become an increasingly large proportion of the population. That is what makes Penny's method of such momentous importance. It is the only one that can legitimately offer a real chance of sustained well-being.

Initially, the best way to explain what Penny has discovered is through her personal experience. So Part One starts with Dorothy's story, from which all the basic SPECAL theories and practices developed. Part Two is wholly practical: it provides a manual for putting the theory into practice, a systematic set of techniques for delivering well-being.[5] Part Three completes the exposition of wraparound care by explaining how to transfer it into a nursing home.

Quite rightly, the British treat the hyperbolic claims of most self-help books with the scepticism that they deserve. Nonetheless, I am going to make one of those bloated-sounding claims: after you have read this book and put it into practice, it really will transform for the better the well-being of both you and the person for whom you care. You must be the judge of whether I am right and there is only one way to find out: get reading!

---

[5] There is support available for readers who are struggling with any aspect of the method at www.special.co.uk. See also www.oliver-james-books.com for further details of relevant work by me. For readers who do not have access to the internet, written communications can be sent to: The SPECAL Centre, Sheep Street, Burford OX18 4LS.

Part One

MAKING SENSE OF DEMENTIA

CHAPTER ONE

Dorothy's Story

Dorothy Johnson was 59 years old when she first noticed insidious changes in her memory, which had been infallible up to then. As an accomplished and competitive Bridge player, she began to experience 'blips' in her sequencing skills at critical points in the game. She would lose track of one significant card and fail to complete strategies that normally would have been guaranteed.

When she mentioned this to her family, she was told that she was taking the game too seriously, but she noticed other problems. She had always maintained a casual approach to the whereabouts of her spectacles, purse, keys or handbag at any particular time. For years it had been a family joke that when it was time to leave the house she would dash to gather these together only at the last minute. But there came a sinister development in this familiar pattern: on occasion she had trouble making any sort of informed guess as to where her handbag might be. She became increasingly convinced that there was something wrong: a brain tumour, perhaps? This suggestion was gently dismissed by the family, who saw only an exaggeration of well-established characteristic traits.

Her husband, Sam, was a distinguished GP. As time passed, he picked up significant signs of memory change. However, he excluded the possibility of an acute condition and openly discouraged any medical investigation. He knew only too well the limitations of what medicine had to offer, but Dorothy persisted that something untoward was going on. Sam reluctantly yielded to her requests for a brain scan and this revealed evidence of substantial, irreversible brain atrophy. In an attempt to protect her from distress, she was not told about this. Rather, she was informed there was no brain tumour and exhorted to make more effort with her memory in future. 'In that case I must be going dotty,' she concluded.

'Nonsense!' came the swift reply from Sam, 'You must just make more effort, that's all.'

He continued to dismiss her concerns, extolling the virtues of various memory aids. Dorothy gamely tried to write everything down but one day sadly enquired of her daughter Penny Garner, 'What is the point of writing lists if I can't remember to read them?' In the car one day, she turned to Penny and said, out of the blue, 'If I turn into one of those dotty old women, you must promise you will put me in a home!' Penny laughed, wondering what on earth she was talking about, but her mother persevered and sounded totally serious, as if it was the single most important request she had made in her life. 'Please promise me. I mean it. You simply must. If I turn into a dotty old woman it will make no sense to leave me at home to interfere with everyone else's life. Put me in a home. I shall be fine, I promise you.' Eventually she extracted a promise from her rather nonplussed daughter and they went on their way to the beach.

Penny was to return to that conversation many times but it was not for several years that she noticed her mother was less able to give the sort of in-depth advice that had been such a feature of their relationship. She simply could not cope with too many details and although hard to separate from her usual patterns, other changes were also taking place. Food shopping had never interested her, unless for a special occasion. Now, endless trips to the shops were required, as each time she returned home without at least one important item she had intended to buy. Never one to exult in domestic tasks, her lack of application to running the home was nonetheless becoming much more pronounced. When the trusty cleaning lady, Mildred, left because of her own family commitments it was soon apparent that Mildred had been protecting Dorothy in many small but significant ways.

Things started to verge on the chaotic. Telephone messages were not relayed – an unheard of occurrence until then – and Sam's medical practice was suffering. Eventually, he announced that he would take early retirement, a decision that horrified Dorothy. She insisted privately to Penny that this would result in a disastrous loss of self-esteem for him. He talked privately to Penny of moving to a smaller, more manageable house. Dorothy was aghast. Surely they had always said they would never move? Dorothy told Penny that she would not be able to cope with the interference of Sam organising the domestic scene if he retired and they moved. Penny talked to each parent in turn, again and again, over several months, and was confused herself as to which one to listen to, which way to turn.

Then Dorothy's GP sent for Penny without telling Sam and delivered a bombshell: that for some years Dorothy had been suffering from a progressive, irreversible form of dementia. The GP told Penny that Sam was fully aware of this but refused to discuss it with anyone. Dementia was not a medical but a management problem. Dorothy was losing her memory, bit by bit, and eventually would lose it entirely. 'We need our memory for everything,' he said. 'Eventually she will forget how to walk, to talk, to eat, and, in the final stages, to breathe.' A silent revolt surged up in Penny: surely there was something that someone could do about it? Then she realized he had not finished. He was adding several other statements which remain etched on Penny's mind to this day: a house move at this stage would be disastrous; it was imperative that she remained where she was until full nursing care was needed, which it undoubtedly would be, but not yet; successful management lay in avoiding confrontation at all times and minimising change to familiar routines.

Penny was stunned by this stark portrait of a situation whose existence, until that moment, she had barely glimpsed, let alone understood. She was reeling with shock about the future and certainly didn't see how she would ever be able to stop her father making the move he was so determined upon. How could she persuade Sam to change his decision without a huge confrontation? It so happened that a tiny cottage had just come on the market only 150 yards down the lane. At least this proximity would preserve a few of Dorothy's daily routines, like walking to the shops, and might leave her some independence from Sam. The cottage proved an acceptable compromise to both parents.

Further advice from the GP followed: Penny should study the movement of a crab, which only moves forward by moving sideways. She must learn to move in that way, not confronting Dorothy with her own dementia, and never challenging her decisions head-on. Dorothy's confidence was the key. The past should be celebrated, not mourned.

After the move from the family home to the cottage occurred, Penny set about following the advice she had been given, to the letter. She made the best of today, but kept to everything she knew Dorothy enjoyed from long ago and limited anything new to a minimum. Dorothy was her old self for much of the time whenever

Penny visited, although Penny was on several occasions left gasping at the enormity of some of her mother's casual remarks. Dorothy said to her one day, 'Isn't it funny? I only ever lose my memory with Daddy. I have no problem at all with anyone else!' Another time, they were standing in the kitchen making mugs of tea. Penny had added the milk and handed Dorothy the milk bottle to replace in the fridge while she carried the tray of tea next door. When Dorothy failed to arrive in the sitting room, Penny popped back to the kitchen. She caught sight of Dorothy contemplating the milk bottle in complete puzzlement. Catching sight of Penny she said, 'Oh, thank goodness you're here! Could you just give me a clue? What am I doing with this?' With Dorothy's help, Penny was beginning to get the hang of what dementia was about.

Together, Penny and Dorothy had a series of adventures, each more zany than the last. On a day out shopping in London, Dorothy decided she'd like a new skirt. In those days the shop assistant used to hover helpfully in the changing room to assist the customer as they tried everything on. As Dorothy slipped off her own skirt to try on the selection of new possibilities, she revealed a second skirt underneath. The expression on the shop assistant's face was priceless. Both skirts were removed without comment and every other one tried on. When Dorothy selected one of her own skirts as the most suitable new one to buy, the shop assistant gulped and Penny beamed, 'Such a good choice – the least expensive of them all.' Dorothy was delighted at the news and promptly put it on. The second of her own skirts also proved helpful, as Penny prevailed upon the baffled assistant to place it in a carrier bag as their new purchase. They left happily discussing how satisfactory it was to pick up a real bargain.

Life with Dorothy was often like living in Alice's Wonderland and Penny would not have missed it for the world. She discovered that one or two routines could be repeated again and again, because Dorothy never seemed to tire of what she enjoyed. The frequent repetition did not bother her. Provided she felt secure, she was able to make her own sense of any situation and then it was just a case of Penny making sure that no one else interfered. Penny herself developed a complete indifference to what other people thought, as long as her mother remained happy. She noticed that when waiting somewhere, such as in the supermarket checkout queue, Dorothy assumed they were at the airport in the duty-free lounge and about to embark on an exciting journey. Provided no one tried to put her straight, they progressed along splendidly, almost without a hitch. Using the ludicrously simple tactic of agreeing with everything Dorothy said worked like a charm and anything else was disastrous. Together, she and Penny lived a happy shambles.

Sam, on the other hand, organised everything in the cottage with military precision and now that he was retired, he devoted his full energy to it. A perfectionist, he could hoover faster and more adroitly than anyone else, so long as no one got in the way. Depending on whose point of view you accepted, Dorothy managed to get in the way incessantly – or was it the hoovering that got in her way? Sam found it virtually impossible to see her perspective on anything. Why pack a suitcase for a flight you aren't taking? He just couldn't get the hang of living with someone with dementia at all.

Dorothy was no longer allowed to drive and her car was sold. Her bank account was closed. She was handed small amounts of pocket money each week by Sam, something that perplexed and annoyed her, and she, in turn, perplexed and annoyed him. The examples of their mutual confusion became depressingly repetitive. Whenever Penny visited, Dorothy explained that she felt completely trapped. Living alone with what appeared to her to be a deranged companion, a volatile situation developed as their lives gradually fell apart.

She was hesitant on the telephone when golf and Bridge friends rang up, usually confused about which was which. Gradually they all gave up. Sam discouraged anyone from dropping in and the old friends began to fade away. With Dorothy now in the cottage all the time, Sam found himself just as trapped as she. The mirroring of each other's situation was truly dreadful. In desperation, Sam became friendly with a new neighbour who felt she must do something to help. Unlike Dorothy, she played neither golf nor Bridge, but kindly offered to take Dorothy to visit some of her own friends for tea while Sam had an afternoon off. As far as Dorothy was concerned, no one there had anything in common with her, and with profound good sense and impeccable manners she politely left within five minutes of arriving. She was promptly recaptured and led back inside by the anxious volunteer neighbour, offered some more tea that she declined, again politely, and again asked to be allowed to leave. And so it went on, week after week, as the neighbour desperately tried to be helpful to Sam, who in the end kept Dorothy at home all the time, refusing to let her go out at all.

Help arrived in the form of Mildred, the much-loved helper from the past who was now persuaded to return to work part-time. As long as Mildred was present in the cottage, there were relatively few problems but she could do nothing about all the other hours of the week when she was not there. Dorothy went down with a severe attack of trigeminal shingles, spent a week in a huge general hospital and on her return home was more at sea than ever. Various drugs were introduced to try and control the situation but Sam soon agreed with the GP that these all made her general condition worse. He said to Penny one day, with tears in his eyes, 'What on earth can I do? I wasn't trained to fail.'

An old friend from Sam's medical days kept in touch. One day the friend rang Penny privately to say he felt that the situation was becoming volatile and potentially quite dangerous. He felt strongly that she should consider moving Dorothy out. Penny was appalled. Then she remembered her promise to her mother all that time ago, to be sure to put her into a home if she ever turned into a 'dotty old woman'. Was she dotty? In a way, yes; in another way, definitely not. What would she have had to say, if only Penny could have asked her? What would she want? Suddenly there was no question. Dorothy had given Penny explicit instructions to do whatever needed doing, indeed Penny had promised to 'do the sensible thing'. With a heavy heart, privately acknowledging that she had Dorothy's consent and accompanied by a curious sense of purpose, Penny began quietly to explore what alternatives there might be to the cottage.

Mildred was deeply concerned at the idea of uprooting Dorothy to somewhere new but agreed a nursing home near Penny's house was the least worst option. Sam could visit Dorothy when he came to stay with Penny. She then tackled Sam about a plan she and Mildred were making for 'separate holidays' for them both.

Penny visited various possible homes willing to countenance confused clients and did her best to erase the details of each from her mind as she drove hurriedly away, in one case moments after entering the front door. Each seemed more indigestible than the last and she could not imagine Dorothy in any of them. Then a friend took Penny to have tea with her grandmother who had moved into a nursing home and seemed to be very happy. The grandmother reminded Penny greatly of her mother: elegant and charming. It was like a genteel, convalescent hotel with flowers in the entrance hall, a properly laid out tea trolley with a selection of sandwiches and cakes. Penny asked to meet the matron, who seemed entirely preoccupied with her ability to pay the fees and her mother's bathroom habits, something that Penny had never considered in such detail before. 'Is she incontinent? I must make it clear that we don't take anyone incontinent here.' Penny hastened to reassure her that Dorothy was fine, incontinence-wise. A bed was almost immediately available, no further questions were asked and within days Penny arrived with Dorothy and her suitcase. Dorothy was swept away by a member of staff. Penny tried to convey a few handy tips about what made her mother tick, but found herself politely ushered out. She went home with fingers firmly crossed and longing to know what was happening.

After three days the matron telephoned. 'Will you kindly come at once! You must remove your mother immediately. How soon can you be here?' Dropping children in every direction, Penny was at the nursing home an hour later, facing the white-faced matron at her desk in the office. 'Your mother is a wanderer!' she declared accusingly. 'Why did you not tell us? You must remove her at once!' Penny asked falteringly what she meant. The matron tersely explained that Dorothy had started exhibiting many instances of unacceptable behaviour within minutes of her arrival, including leaving her chair during tea. Apparently Dorothy had slipped out of the door while no one was looking and had set off down the drive. When recaptured by a member of staff coming on duty, Dorothy had explained that she was 'going shopping'. The matron had personally taken time to explain to Dorothy that there were no shops in the vicinity and that she must remain in her seat at all times. Dorothy deliberately flouted instructions, setting off again several times and always with the same explanation when recaptured. She was going shopping. The matron explained in a starched voice that people like her mother were 'wanderers' and had no place in nursing homes. Where, then, Penny asked nervously, did they belong? The matron gave her a pitying look, wrote out a few words on a piece of scrap paper and passed it across the desk. As she did so she rang a bell and ordered Dorothy and her luggage to be sent down to the front hall. Penny stuffed the scrap of paper in her pocket as she was frogmarched along to wait for her. Dorothy eventually arrived, looking somewhat perplexed, and mother and daughter set off for home where Dorothy resumed life with an ever more exhausted Sam.

Penny and Mildred between them restored some sort of equilibrium to the household and Penny returned to her own home over a hundred miles away. She checked the scrap of paper and was relieved to find the address she had been given was nearby. It turned out to be a large-ish country house with various makeshift extensions, for the most part consisting of corrugated plastic and with an atmosphere reminiscent of Fawlty Towers. She was ushered into a tiny office where she found, sitting behind a desk piled precariously high with papers, an eccentric character referred to with some reverence as 'The Professor' by the staff. He greeted her with a keenly observant look. 'Welcome!' he said, with obvious delight at the sight of a new arrival in his office, 'And what can we do for you?' Over the next half hour they chatted about her plight and his life's work, and how the two might come together to their mutual advantage.

During the course of the conversation there was a constant stream of visitors popping their heads around the door seeking information. A nurse in search of a missing bishop, a postman delivering what appeared to be paper napkins and an opera singer who had lost all her teeth and most of her clothes. All were greeted with politeness and deference by The Professor, and seemed happy with various explanations that Penny found obscure. The distinction between patients and staff was curiously blurred. She asked what happened to 'wanderers' here. She was immediately assured that the staff were under strict instructions to allow every new resident to do exactly what they wanted for the first three days and nights following their arrival at the home. If they wanted baths in the middle of the night, or meals every five minutes, or walks to the next county, their wish was never denied. After the first 72 hours of unconditional acceptance of whatever they wished to do, no one was ever a bit of trouble again. It was a time-honoured ritual that he had learned paid off in a remarkable way.

Dorothy moved in the following week. Penny was encouraged to drop in at any time of the day or night. Dorothy spent the first few days mainly in and out of the kitchen and the office, checking that the cook was happy, that the laundry was sorted and that proper travel arrangements were in place for her impending departure. Her enquiries were treated with respect and she graciously accepted the expressions of thanks that flowed from the staff. Gradually she moved about less, although she maintained an interest in the activities of the kitchen. Penny would arrive as inconspicuously as possible, in order to catch a fly-on-the-wall glimpse of her mother's life in the home. Dorothy was usually contentedly busy, but would stop for a cup of tea if encouraged by the staff. She and Penny would sit alongside each other in the residents' lounge, a crowded, dingy room with torn lino on the floor, surrounded by people in varying states of animation and decrepitude. Dorothy would talk in an excited way about travel arrangements and as they discussed possible scenarios, Penny would begin to see the room through her eyes. At times, it was an overcrowded airport departure lounge and their companions were fellow tour members; at others, it was a large party of friends that Dorothy was attentively hosting; on another, it was a medical convention which was clearly boring her rigid.

Over the next four years Dorothy's mental prowess declined. As her English vocabulary became increasingly vague she used French words instead, having lived in France as a child. She and a Moroccan cleaner at the home exchanged pleasantries right up to the end of her life, based on a few simple, shared phrases which eventually turned into friendly nods and a wave of the hand.

When she visited, Penny made it a rule to stay only long enough to find out whether life was acceptable. It seemed crucial to ask the question, 'Is everything all right, Mum?' and to receive the flickering, reassuring nod in response. The process of making sufficient contact to obtain an answer was like fiddling with a faulty electric plug that would only connect to the mains socket in a random, intermittent way. The fiddling had to be done by reaching out with the eyes, quietly murmuring and touching her mother's hand as if there were all the time in the world. Sometimes Penny fiddled for hours and at others it only took a moment or two to make the connection. Sooner or later Dorothy would give the all-important 'I'm okay' nod, even if in later life this was only with the eyes. The sense of relaxation as they engaged was palpable. Penny would sit back in her chair while Dorothy resumed her former activity, whatever that might have been. In the early years at the home that would involve pottering off to the kitchen to supervise. In later years Dorothy would resume a gentle doze in her chair. Penny would take the opportunity to slip quietly away, seeking out a member of staff to watch over Dorothy as she left.

One day, however, Penny ran into a real problem. She had been at the home for hours, sitting alongside Dorothy, fiddling, as it were, with the plug, without getting any response. It was time for her to pick the children up from school. Without the reassurance that all was well, she felt she could not leave and did the only thing she could think of. She telephoned a friend to pick up the children so she could stay. Observing her carefully throughout the evening, it eventually became clear that Dorothy had a throat infection and was running a temperature. Penny discussed the situation with the staff and Dorothy was put on a course of antibiotics, tucked up in bed and was soon on the road to recovery. Penny realised her mother had communicated in the only way she could: by withholding communication altogether.

This situation repeated itself on three further occasions over the next few years, and each time Penny was able to establish that Dorothy was physically unwell. By remaining by her side, Penny had the luxury of open-ended time in which to pick up further clues as to what precisely was wrong.

Otherwise, Penny was unfailingly rewarded with a connection, however brief, which made clear that Dorothy was fundamentally okay. Very occasionally, she would reveal startlingly longer moments of lucidity, as if to remind Penny that she could take nothing for granted about her apparent state of cognitive decline. It was as if, while appearing to doze, she had actually been listening all the time.

There were several chaotic incidents in the nursing home as Dorothy settled in, including the day when she created a new system of storage in the linen cupboard. Each episode was greeted with politeness from the staff and Dorothy sailed serenely on. It was truly an eccentric place. The clothes the residents wore were unusual and often remarkably few. Penny became quite used to seeing Dorothy in an unaccustomed combination of items, rarely her own, and all had suffered the dire consequences of the antiquated and unreliable laundry system. Any stockings – and sometimes several – were invariably around her ankles and her hair was in need of a good brush. There were aspects of the physical environment that were dire but the emotional well-being of the residents was unmistakably and consistently strong.

Whenever Sam came to stay, Penny would hurry over to the nursing home on her own, allowing at least an hour to restore Dorothy to something like a normal appearance before bringing her to meet him. These encounters were increasingly stressful for everyone, particularly Sam, who never stopped asking Dorothy questions and always drew attention to any slight deficit in her overall appearance. Penny never allowed him to enter the nursing home, as she was terrified he would have Dorothy removed on the spot. In due course she suggested to Sam that Dorothy not come during his visits and with huge relief, mixed with a comparable amount of guilt, he no longer saw Dorothy at all. Penny found the whole situation most challenging but had no doubt whatsoever that this was the sensible path. Dorothy was saved any trauma and Sam returned home less depressed once the near-intolerable meetings no longer took place.

Finally, after nearly four years in the nursing home, Dorothy began to slip away. The first sign of change was another withholding of communication that led to Penny, yet again, needing to find out what was wrong. Her brother was over from South Africa for a rare visit, so the family had gathered together at the nursing home for a reunion. This time Dorothy had a virulent mouth infection which was spreading. The family identified the problem, found a straw for her to drink through and established ways of helping her to eat less painfully. Dorothy tuned in and sat serenely on the chair in her room, holding her hands out to Penny's middle daughter in the way Penny knew so well. 'Come and kiss me goodbye,' she said, and her little granddaughter led the procession of affectionate farewells.

Dorothy was flooded with antibiotics, but it was now too late. She never spoke again. She declined steadily over the succeeding five days and by the next weekend Penny was over at the home, sitting beside her mother for the remaining 37 hours of her life. Those hours are among Penny's most precious memories. She left Dorothy's side only three times and only for moments. Penny recalls that she gained, then, more information about what life is all about than at any other time either before or since. There were extraordinary moments, both mystically untrammelled by time and yet intensely immediate in their impact. The most peaceful one came at the end, after what seemed like a final, frenetic flurry. Penny had the impression of a bird that was trying to escape the room, repeatedly flying towards the closed window and fluttering against it in an ever more frantic attempt to reach the freedom of the open space beyond. It was as if there was no handle to open the window and Penny sat helplessly, wondering what to do, feeling powerless to intervene in any useful way. She felt sure she would see the bird drop with exhaustion and quietly expire on the carpet beneath the window. But then, as if an unseen hand turned the handle just as the bird made a final desperate attempt, the window opened and the bird sailed through, onward and upward and away to the horizon beyond, faster than the speed of light.

As Penny drove away from the home shortly after 5 a.m. she vowed that one day, goodness knows how or when, she would live to see the day when all carers would share the in-depth understanding of dementia that she had been given by Dorothy. Above all she wanted to put right the fact that she had never been able to share her knowledge with Sam. She knew that she had been given a blueprint, an instruction book, a new pair of glasses, a job to do, a task to fulfil. She knew it would take a long time but she also had a sense of peaceful conviction. As she drove along the straight stretch of road before descending the hill that led to her house, the words of the mediaeval mystic, Dame Julian of Norwich, floated through her mind: 'All shall be well, and all shall be well, and all manner of thing shall be well.'

CHAPTER TWO

Getting Started

Dorothy's death occurred at the end of 1984 but it was to be some years before the work of making 'all well' commenced. Starting from scratch, even if Penny Garner had had more qualifications than a secretarial training and not had responsibility for three young daughters, developing a completely new way of managing people with dementia would have been daunting. It was not until 1990 that she finally clicked into action. She called her local Alzheimer's Society and got an immediate response: they needed someone to go to a meeting at her local community hospital in Burford just a few days later. Funds had recently become available to modernise the existing Day Unit and one day a week had been set aside for the 'elderly mentally ill' – which really meant people with dementia – with the object of giving their carers a break. The day selected was Friday.

From the moment when the first patient walked in it was abundantly clear that Penny knew how to deal with him. She instantly recognised her mother's ailment and made a connection. Since he was called Paddy, she professed a love of Ireland and, digging around in her memory for something Irish, she came up with dancing and the Irish jig. Within 10 minutes they were chatting with great animation; within 20, he was showing her the steps as they reeled around the room.

Paddy also came to the Day Unit on days other than Friday. Although he would be in the same room, the social environment was so different that he would behave quite differently. In fact, he had been sent to Penny as the most troublesome person the staff had ever known and they were relieved to get shot of him in her direction on at least one day of the week.

Having worked as a master baker, he tended to head for the kitchen and would sometimes pick up knives. With no knowledge of his former profession, the staff on days other than Friday were terrified. He was totally disruptive, spending his time wanting to get home, plagued by worrying questions: Where was his wife? Why was he here? Why were they stopping him going home? Their responses would come back: 'Your wife is not here because she's having a rest'; 'You aren't at home because your wife's not at home, so you can't be either.' To this latter explanation he would respond, 'Do you seriously mean that my wife would not be happy that I was at home on my own?' Finally, inexorably, going down that line long enough, the carers found themselves saying, 'I'm sorry Paddy, you've just gotta stay here', at which point he would turn round and say 'I'm sorry, but I am actually leaving, right now', and the scene was set for big trouble. By contrast, when he came on a Friday, within 30 seconds of seeing Penny he was with someone he had 'known for years' and was thrilled to meet. He was happy to sit down calmly, have a cup of coffee and then find he could help her with her Irish reeling. The awkward questions did not arise.

If Penny's first strategy was to find a common interest, the second was never to ask questions. Questioning almost invariably entailed a reminder that memory was impaired, that information was missing. She would never ask, 'How was your journey?' or 'How did you get here?' or any other direct question, as an opening gambit. With Paddy it was a case of assuming from his name that he was Irish and then, 'How riveting, my mother lived in Ireland for a time' to which he replied, 'Which part?' What she wanted was them asking the questions. Give her someone new with dementia, then or now, and using this questionless technique she would expect to be having an animated conversation within 30 seconds. She also knew then not to assume any knowledge of the recent past – that was 'dead ground and ridiculous'. It was this understanding that made her react so assertively when other people would opine that the mind of a person with dementia is 'absolutely shot'. She would say firmly, 'No it's not. It's only shot in terms of what's just happened. But memories from long ago are still there. Surely anyone can see that?'

While Penny and her colleagues got better and better at what they did, they had no success in transferring their achievements to Paddy's home. His wife got ever more tired, and she would tell them how awful it was. Penny tried to convey something of his positive mood at the unit but that did not help at all. His wife was saying he was antagonistic and potentially violent, and that her beloved husband of yesteryear was gone. Telling her that he was happy when not with her was hardly a boost and she became severely upset and depressed.

In due course it became horrendous. The community psychiatric nurse was called in and Paddy was admitted to a nursing home. On the very first day he went into its kitchen in search of his baker's workplace. Equipped with a knife, he was looking for a loaf to cut when the cook came in and had a fit. She saw a madman about to stab her to death, not a baker wanting to start work. Emergency buttons were pressed and he was taken away to a secure mental unit. Penny visited him there a couple of times and found she could still wake him from his nightmare existence and elicit an Irish smile. But it was only a matter of months before she was informed of his death.

An octogenarian called Alice was the first person to whom Penny succeeded in delivering lifelong well-being. Alice's husband, Tim, had been providing devoted care for seven years. When Penny first visited them at their cottage, Alice's immediate memory span was about 10 seconds. She had no record in her brain of the facts of what had happened only moments before, such as Penny arriving and being introduced, or discussions about a cup of tea. Yet Alice's memories of times past were still there. She remembered her ancient boxer dog, to whom she was visibly attached, and knew her way around the cottage.

Knee-high-to-a-grasshopper, she was a beaky little person, very sharp, bright-eyed, suspicious and keen to suss out who Penny was and what she was up to. When Penny tried to be encouraging by saying Alice looked well, she noticed a quizzical look in return – why was someone Alice did not know trying to compliment her?

A conventional psychiatrist might have misinterpreted this as paranoia but Penny understood the rationale. During one of her visits to the cottage a meter man called, explaining what he needed to do. Alice showed him the meter in the kitchen and returned to the tea party. Moments later, Alice heard some hammering, leaped up from her chair and went into the hall to investigate. She caught sight of a complete stranger in her kitchen. She reacted with 'Out! What are you doing here?', assuming the meter man was a thief. That was neither paranoid nor delusional, simply that she had no idea why this peculiar person was in her house, a reaction any of us might have if we were confronting a complete stranger.

By Penny's third visit for tea, she had begun to gather more background information about what made Alice tick. While Tim was out of the room for a short while, Penny employed a technique she had already developed for putting patients at ease and raising their confidence in the Day Unit: she acted the part of someone whose memory is less than perfect, saying things like 'Oh dear, sometimes I almost forget my own name!' With an eager look, Alice immediately asked if she had a problem with her memory and she replied 'Mine's not too bad, but my *mother*, she really had a terrible problem. She had an absolutely hopeless memory!' Alice asked more about Dorothy and so, unwittingly, about herself. Given her predicament, she was riveted as Penny explained that there was excellent news because Dorothy had managed brilliantly, despite her poor memory. Dementia was not necessarily bad news and Penny was able to reassure Alice that very specialised help was now available, right there in Burford.

Alice had always been fiercely independent and disliked feeling disempowered by her illness, more than anything else. She dealt with her increasingly heavy dependence on her husband by describing Tim as her servant and, to add insult to injury, as an inadequate one. Not surprisingly, Tim was finding this difficult – 'I'm hanging on by my fingertips' – and viewed the future bleakly. Caring for his wife was wrecking his life, upsetting him and making him feel like a failure for being unable to be a more successful carer. His account of her was of someone who was completely crazy and driving him mad, an impossible woman. It was clear that Alice was a shadow of her former self, with rock-bottom confidence, fearful of being left alone even while Tim went off to the loo, and refusing to leave the house; yet also, she had become an autocrat who felt no compunction in ordering him around all over the place.

As Penny was to find in so many subsequent cases, there were large discrepancies between the person the spouse or offspring knows, the one Penny meets and the person's account of themselves. From her experience with Dorothy, Penny expected that Alice would know she had a problem and sure enough, at that first meeting, Alice told her that if she met her again she would not recognise her because of 'a problem with my memory'. However, she only said this when her husband was not in the room and Tim told Penny later that he did not believe his wife knew she was ill.

Penny made repeated brief visits to the cottage and while Alice appeared to have no factual memory of their previous meetings, she became increasingly comfortable in Penny's company, which suggested that some feelings had been stored. Alice might not be able to put a name to Penny's face but positive feelings were associated with it.

It emerged that Alice had played the card game of Contract Bridge to a very high standard. Improbably, Penny decided to build on this experience – improbably, because anyone who has ever played the game will tell you that someone who can only remember events from 10 seconds ago would be peculiarly ill-equipped to play. Playing Bridge with dementia was as counter-intuitive as encouraging a deaf person to be a telephone operator using a normal phone, or someone who is blind to seek employment as an air traffic controller without any aids.

Penny wanted to use Bridge to give Alice the sense that she was on familiar ground, to provide a context. Penny knew it would not be exactly the same as the usual game but perhaps it would seem so to Alice if she could draw on her experiences from a long time ago, well before dementia struck. Penny knew Alice was highly knowledgeable on the subject. The idea came from looking after Dorothy.

Penny had often thought of Dorothy as like a person watching a video in which the pictures and the words did not match. Dorothy had been an eager and adventurous traveller, so that going on trips had been an important, happy part of her life. After she developed dementia, when in a busy room, she could believe she was waiting for a plane in the departure lounge at Heathrow. Whenever this belief was challenged, she would have a problem. While she was waiting for a plane, she would suddenly find herself surrounded by people who were speaking as if they were quite somewhere else, engaged in a different activity. She was seeing one narrative but hearing another, a most confusing discontinuity.

Over the years working at Burford, Penny saw many cases where this caused major problems for both patients and staff. For example, Penny was invited to visit a local mental health hospital to see if she could solve a troublesome problem. The staff believed one of their patients, Bill, might die unless they could get him to drink, but he refused any liquids. Penny had met Bill some time ago during one of his stays in Burford Hospital. When Penny learned which anti-psychotic pills they were now giving him, she guessed that he believed he was being poisoned. In spite of her lay status, she already knew that this particular medication often caused severe problems. Among the side effects listed on Bill's packet were 'hallucinations' (which was what the staff told Penny that they hoped the drug would treat), 'Parkinsonism' (trembles that were now making him unsteady on his feet), as well as 'drowsiness' and 'claustrophobia'. She figured that his brain was telling him he was being poisoned so he had decided not to drink anything, but she also knew that he loved going down to the pub. To test her theory, Penny took along a colleague and a few beer tankards later that day. The two of them perched on stools at a conveniently high reception desk, as if it were a bar, and carried on for all

the world as if they were in the pub. The receptionist appeared somewhat put out but received a warning look from Penny not to comment.
Sure enough, Bill soon stumbled across to join them; the conversation
was already on his favourite topic, snooker, and, secure that he would
not be ingesting pill-infested liquid, he happily gave up his self-
dehydration. Once Penny had got the picture to fit with the sound Bill
was fine and Penny hoped to use Bridge to do the same for Alice.

Over the course of her visits to Alice's cottage Penny
repeatedly mentioned a Bridge Club she was setting up for
beginners. Penny watched Alice closely and observed that she was
drawn into the idea each time the subject was brought up. Alice
had always approved of people taking up the game, keen to
encourage them. She had clear memories of just how difficult she
had found it when she had first started and how important
confidence is at that stage for anyone.

Although Penny sensed that she was gaining consent from Alice
to involve her in some sort of Bridge activity, she also knew that she
would have to tread carefully. Dorothy had taught her that in seconds
a blunder would cause a total transformation. Dorothy's face could
turn from a bright, happy look to become grey and expressionless
when confronted by an incomprehensible situation: the pictures with
the wrong soundtrack. Creating a continuity of common
understanding in which the emotional killers were eradicated and
there were only vivifiers was the real game here.

The first time they played, Alice was comfortable so long as
there was a tremendous amount of social 'scaffolding' to keep her in
touch with normal life within the context of Bridge. The most
important enlivener was the partaking of tea, rather than the Bridge
itself. Much of the time was taken up distributing the cups and
pouring and, because this was tea in the context of Bridge, Alice

made the connection with a familiar, pleasing experience that she engaged in with confidence.

When Alice's Bridge moved to the Friday Group, Penny soon discovered that a crushed-velvet tablecloth was all that was required to carry the message to Alice that she was in a Bridge-playing environment, and as such she was happy to settle down at any table. The scorers, the playing cards or the players did not carry the same message but as soon as the appropriate Bridge cloth was on a table, Alice would head in that direction, seeming to think that she was about to play or had just done so. Penny proved this to herself by experiments. She tried just the cards, just the score card, just four people sitting round a square table but it was only the cloth which provided sure confirmation to Alice of 'Bridge'. It also helped to adopt her particular pet phrases for different aspects of the game, in that she clearly preferred, 'Whose go is it?' rather than, 'Who's the dealer?' and if everyone used Alice's precise form of words it greatly contributed to the patina of normality. The challenge for Penny was to stay constantly alert to any signs that Alice was losing connection with her old lines.

On the very first occasion at the cottage when Penny had actually got out the cards, Alice looked momentarily terrified and Penny suddenly feared that the whole afternoon was going to turn into a nightmare. In desperation, she deliberately dropped the pack on the floor, which worked like a spell. Instantly, Alice was in control and the competent one: 'Stupid child, dear, dear, dear,' she tutted. Transformed into the host with the most, she helped pick them up, with Penny in the role of the ham-fisted, apologetic person needing sorting out, like the cards. With confidence happily restored, Alice soon demonstrated that she still knew how to shuffle the pack, to deal and to organise her hand.

During the game Alice needed constant reminders of what was happening. This was provided by Penny forming a 'we-relationship' with her, in which they were both helping two novice players along. She would occasionally send Alice a conspiratorial look across the table, raising her eyebrows as if to say, 'Goodness me, aren't these other two slow!' Alice was quick to respond in a similar style. Whenever Alice paused and looked as if she had lost track, Penny would comment, 'Now, let's see, I think it must be their turn.' She closely monitored Alice to provide continuity of narrative. As soon as she knew that Alice had become disorientated, or was about to be, not only was Penny able to act but she had a technique for doing so which reversed the true position regarding who had lost the plot. Once Alice received a subtle cue, she knew it was her turn and had no difficulty in performing her role, albeit that the bid she made might be at variance with what had gone before. If you think of her as like an actor in a play, where all the other performers are suddenly speaking lines from a different script, you can understand both how terrifying it would be to realise this had happened and how relieving to get a prompt which allows it all to make instant sense again.

Following this success, Penny asked Tim to bring Alice over to the Bridge Club she had actually set up in her own village. All members, many of them comparative novices, were given help in understanding the play within the play entailing Alice. On one occasion, a player counted Alice's tricks for her, as Alice seemed to be getting her sums wrong. This led to one of Alice's familiar piercing looks, since it was breaching Bridge protocol and seemed to be treating her like a beginner. Sustaining a good-natured and non-competitive form of the game was crucial and as the novices improved, Alice recovered many of her past skills.

In some ways, the three other players were subtly fostering an illusion that normal play was in progress, with Alice helping out some less good players. In one sense that is what was happening; in another, they were acting out roles, ignoring any occasions on which Alice broke basic rules and pretending as if the game was progressing in the usual fashion, which it often was not. They did nothing to indicate to Alice that she was anything other than an experienced player and they were careful to imply that if anyone was struggling, it was them, not her. This was not a simple matter of crude deception, in which they deliberately misled her towards a delusion. Rather, it was a case of taking up clues from her as to who she felt herself to be in that moment and what she assumed she was doing. Alice had certainly been an experienced player and it was this person that, in their company, she often continued to be. So long as they went to considerable lengths to do nothing to disturb the sense she was making of her surroundings, her pictures and soundtrack matched.

Penny's great insight was that building upon a real memory is completely different from the encouragement of a delusion. Had Alice never played Bridge or only done so badly it would have been nurturing delusion to plant the idea that she had once been brilliant and still was. Penny was not doing that at all. Alice rightly believed herself to possess great Bridge experience, and Penny was skilfully protecting her from information that contradicted the illusion that she could play Bridge today exactly as she had in the past. If Alice had suffered an actual delusion, such as that she was Queen Victoria or the Virgin Mary, it would have been inappropriate to have encouraged these beliefs. Penny's unique clinical innovation was to spot the benign potential of systematically supporting the re-experience of long-term memories: once an experienced Bridge player, always an experienced Bridge player.

Throughout the nineties Penny worked with over one hundred

hospital patients. When she was asked to explain her work, she was frequently accused of being untruthful to clients, of fostering lunacy and unethical practices. This misunderstood her main point: that she was not planting false memories or supporting delusions, she was nurturing the rich and immutable truth of the person's actual past experiences and achievements, stored long before the dementia. The illusion was in the conflation of the past and the present. Allowing this (acting as if Alice was just as capable as ever), rather than correcting it (pointing to shortcomings in the way she played Bridge), enabled Alice to make sense of the present in terms of her past. Given this help, her insights into the game were as great as they always had been.

Alice really had been a top Bridge player, whereas no schizophrenic ever was Queen Victoria. The real queen never suffered from psychosis but suppose she had developed dementia and was provided with care that fitted in comfortably with her pre-dementia experience of being the monarch? Supporting that idea would be completely different from encouraging a modern patient who thinks they are or were Queen Victoria.

Of course, the Bridge was not all plain sailing. There were several occasions when a friendly game had just started in the Day Unit, when Alice would suddenly decide that she had to get home to feed her beloved boxer dog. She would rise politely from the table, explaining graciously but firmly that she would have to leave. Checking pockets for her key, she would say goodbye and leave the hospital on foot. If Penny was unable to dissuade her from doing this, she simply followed behind at a discreet distance as Alice proceeded to her cottage a quarter of a mile away on the other side of the High Street. The first time it happened Penny was worried that Alice might walk under a bus but was fascinated to observe how drivers seemed to intuit from her confident gait and focused demeanour that she was no average pedestrian, and automatically gave way to her. On the many occasions that Penny followed, Alice never came to harm, arriving safely home. Penny would allow Alice a few minutes to settle in before ringing the bell. When Alice opened the door, Penny said 'Hello Alice. I'm sorry I'm a bit late for the Bridge.' Having no knowledge that she had been playing only five minutes before, Alice would reply, 'Good Lord, are we playing Bridge?' and then, 'Would you like a cup of tea?' Penny would decline politely and explain they were needed to help with the novice players. Alice then shut up the cottage and they went to the hospital, where they would be welcomed by the other players still seated at the table, as if they had just arrived for the first time.

At numerous points during this sequence, a catastrophic collapse of Alice's confidence could have occurred. As she moved from her role of Bridge Player to Dog Owner her reality needed to be sustained. The danger to her confidence was one that would be every bit as great for me if someone were to enter this room now and say 'I know you think you are writing a book about dementia but in fact you are a policeman' or if someone were to interrupt you now and say 'It's time to stop playing tennis', when in fact you are reading these words in this book. If anyone had challenged Alice's autonomous right to leave the hospital at the time of her choosing, it would have rammed home that she was a vulnerable person not in control of her own life. The images would immediately have been at variance with the soundtrack. If Penny had suggested she accompany her to her cottage rather than tracking her, Alice would be thinking 'I don't need someone to walk me home' and would have begun to question why on earth such a warden was necessary. If, on arriving at her cottage or when they returned to the unit, Penny had attempted to remind her of the fact that they had just been playing Bridge, it would have totally thrown her: since she had no stored memory of having just played, it would have seemed completely weird that someone was telling her she had been playing only a few minutes ago.

As time went by, most of Alice's waking life revolved around Bridge. Penny created a loop for her in which a large part of every day consisted of waiting to play, playing, having tea while playing, recovering from having played and discussing plans for playing tomorrow – like a happy version of the film *Groundhog Day*. This made a huge contrast to the deeply suspicious, severely anxious, disempowered autocrat whom Penny had first met some years earlier. Penny learned that you cannot succeed with someone with dementia unless you protect them from all the disastrous experiential roads down which they can so easily travel.

It may be seen that Penny had to acquire a sophisticated understanding of precisely which of Alice's roles were active at any single moment in order to keep these balls in the air. Penny is exceptionally gifted in this art, a mistress of diplomacy, ingenious and flexible in devising benign ways to avoid catastrophic breakdowns of the illusion. Many people have assumed that because the inventor of SPECAL is so good at it, only she could provide this kind of care. However, this turned out not to be so, although it took many years for her to learn how to pass the skills on.

The most important legacy of Penny's work over a period of 10 years alongside the hospital staff, was to liken the illness to a photograph album. That analogy enabled her to teach her clinical methods to many hundreds of grateful clinicians and carers, and you need to understand the idea before you can proceed to the practical techniques described in Part Two.

CHAPTER THREE

The Photograph Album

Penny Garner uses an analogy between our memory and a photograph album to illustrate her view of how memory works.[6] Think of the album as the place where each new memory is stored. The photographs represent individual memories. The ones on the latest pages are the most recent, the photos near the beginning of the album are the oldest.

When awake, we keep our album open on today's page, the 'here and now'. We glance constantly at these latest photographs as we seek to make sense of what we are doing, where we are and who we are with. Sometimes we need to leaf back through recent pages, to seek out further information. Only comparatively rarely do we turn to pages much further back in our album.

Using our album is as fundamental to our mental existence, as breathing is to our physical existence. We take it for granted, it happens automatically and it is a critical component of our identity. It enables us to know what's what at every waking moment.

As we age, our faculties become less efficient and the actual

[6] Garner, P., 'The SPECAL Photograph Album', 2008, Third Edition, Burford, Oxfordshire.

process of consulting our album slows. After the age of 50, we tend to take longer to find photographs that we know to be there. We become aware of this reduction in our speed of retrieval, and therefore, our efficiency (although we may prefer not to dwell on it). In healthy people, despite ageing, the only change relates to the speed and confidence with which we consult our album.

When a memory is stored normally in the album, there are two components. First, there are the facts of the picture. For example, right now, I have lots of images of myself sitting in my office at my computer looking at this screen. Secondly, there are the emotions associated with the facts, such as feeling tired or bored or excited by the work I am doing at this moment. Penny has divided the feelings up, quite simply, into those that are acceptable (characterised as green) and those that are, in stark contrast, wholly unacceptable (characterised as red).

When dementia begins, a single, striking change happens in what gets stored: the factual content is not registered, only the feelings. Hence, if I were developing dementia I might fail to store the fact that I have just written about the distinction between facts and feelings, only left with the feeling of satisfaction that I have been describing something but unclear as to exactly what. When this starts happening, Penny describes the dementia-induced feelings-only, fact-free photographs as 'blanks'.

When the blanks first start coming they are unlikely to cause any problems. They represent only a split-second loss of factual information of what has just happened. However, as the number of blanks increase, the person finds themselves with more and more recent pages in their album where potentially crucial facts are missing. It's not at all the case that the new factual information has been forgotten, either temporarily or otherwise – *it has not entered the album in the first place.* In due course, the person will find themselves unable to ignore or conceal from others the fact that they are missing the information that they need to make sense of what they are currently doing. Sooner or later, it leads to big trouble. Penny provides a telling example.

Chatting at the breakfast table, Arthur asks Dolly if she will post a letter for him. Dolly knows how much Arthur has missed his secretary since his retirement and realises that a wife makes a very poor one. Planning to be really efficient, Dolly tucks the letter carefully in a secure pocket of her handbag. However, she has dementia and this letter conversation enters her album as a feelings-only blank. For Dolly, once that particular exchange has finished, factually it is as if it had never taken place.

At supper, Arthur asks Dolly if she posted his letter. Dolly checks back in her album, looking for the information she requires. Letter? What letter? There's nothing in Dolly's album about a discussion about a letter at breakfast this morning. So Dolly says that she didn't post a letter because there was none to post. Arthur disagrees, insisting there was. He says he can clearly remember the entire conversation. Dolly searches again but still finds nothing. As tactfully as she can, she explains to Arthur that he is wrong. He gets quite angry. He doesn't like Dolly arguing with him, particularly when he knows he's right. Finding her attitude patronising and difficult, he challenges her again. Meanwhile, Dolly finds *his* attitude totally extraordinary and becomes concerned that he is perhaps ill in some way.

In terms of the analogy, Dolly and Arthur are each consulting their own albums, expecting the photographs (facts) to tally. When this does not happen, they assume that the other must be wrong. They expect that closer inspection of their photographs will lead to agreement about the matters under discussion. On this occasion, though, however much they consult their albums, they will find conflicting information that worries and confuses them both.

Arthur insists that Dolly check a particular pocket of her handbag. He says that he remembers exactly where she put the letter. After all, he can see the relevant photographs quite clearly in his own album. Dolly tells him he is mistaken and they begin to argue. Furious at his persistence, Dolly fetches her handbag and opens it to show him that there is no letter. Arthur tells her exactly which compartment to look in and she finds a letter . . . apparently placed there by her earlier in the day, just as he claimed. How could this be? Dolly's heart misses a beat and she is filled with panic. She begins to search once more, again fruitlessly, for information that she now knows beyond any doubt that she ought to be able to find in her album, but which is just not there.

There can be no process of 'remembering' the breakfast conversation because she cannot retrieve information that was not stored in the first place. Dolly has been confronted with clear evidence of a blank that she knew nothing about previously. A serious threat to her emotional well-being has arisen. As she contemplates the new and strange situation an unbearable panic develops on a scale she has never known before. Another person, her husband, has facts about her recent activity in his album that should also be in hers. She had no idea of this until he pointed it out, but now she is fully aware. Massive ill-being follows as she considers what other information she may, unknowingly, have failed to store. She realises that she may never know how many other times this has happened. Meanwhile, Arthur has no idea of what she is now going through.

Penny denotes the state of panic and distress as a 'red'. It is a wholly unacceptable feeling of ill-being, normally (in the absence of dementia) restricted to highly traumatic, relatively rare events, such as hearing of the sudden death of a close relative or another shocking experience. The supper conversation during which the previously unknown blank has been uncovered is a red. It will now be stored as a new photograph in Dolly's album. Since the supper experience is supremely traumatic, as all reds invariably are, Dolly's confidence is severely undermined and a sense of profoundly disturbing distress is generated and stored.

It is all too easy to see from this simple incident how dementia causes major unhappiness for sufferers and tremendous turbulence in relationships with family and friends. But there is worse to come. Unless Penny's kind of care can be provided, as Dolly's dementia progresses there will be a growing number of pages in her photograph album that not only contain reds but are now increasingly blank. To be confronted by a series of red blanks is a nightmare that no person without dementia can fully appreciate – a series of photographs containing wholly unacceptable feelings and entirely devoid of facts to explain where such feelings have come from. As time goes by, Dolly has virtually no full photographs of recent experiences and an intolerably high proportion of red blanks. She is in danger of living out her life in a place as red as hell. And that may, and often does, go on for many years. Small wonder that so many people like Dolly eventually decide to close their album altogether in order to escape the reds.

Most people have very few reds in their life and red is always associated with trauma of some sort. However, the experience of uncovering a red *blank* is particularly horrendous and specific to dementia. Uncovering a red blank provides another red blank and yet another, and the retained feelings of knowing that you are panicked out of your mind and yet have no knowledge why, is more hideous, by far, than knowing the actual facts.

The album analogy helps to explain why dementia is so uniquely ghastly. Without the right help, the person with dementia will be confronted with clear evidence that they lack very recent information about themselves. Unless their distress is attended to using the methods outlined in Part Two, sooner or later their panic is stored as a red blank. For instance, they may not know how they travelled to where they are now standing or sitting, unable to access information that can tell them whether they came by car or walked. This is a strange, new and quite extraordinary situation that, unless they can sort it out, is increasingly likely to induce a disastrous sense of a loss of control. They have no way of avoiding it, they are unlikely to be able to address it on their own and in the usual situation, no one has a remedy.

Penny describes this situation of becoming trapped in a continuous run of red blanks as 'negative ribboning'. One red blank repeatedly gives rise to another and the ribbon that enters the album becomes the unacceptable norm. Exactly like anyone faced with evidence that something is catastrophically wrong, the person with dementia wants urgently to put it right. Unfortunately, lack of relevant data hampers planning and execution of remedial action. They have not lost their reason and in seeking a solution are acting rationally, even though others may view their exertions as incomprehensible, irrational or unjustified, and dismiss them as mad or meaningless. The person only knows that there is red in their album that they must address as a matter of urgency. With no solution, they become trapped in a negative vortex of inescapable panic.

To make sense of it, they search frantically back through their album to seek out an old, intact red (unacceptable feeling) in the early pages. They are looking for a previously resolved traumatic event that they would otherwise normally leave well alone. They seize on this red with a sense of profound relief that at last they have found some distressing facts on which they can now act to address their current panic. But the relief is short-lived, for when they do find an old, intact red and begin to act on it, they are almost bound to be impeded by other people who have no idea what they are up to. The old red photograph which they have located becomes both the explanation for their current distress and the catalyst for action, but it is also completely out of sync with the current experiences of everyone else around them.

For example, suppose they leaf back to a red photograph of a favourite dog that was run over 30 years before. They need to find their children to protect them from too much sadness; they need to bury the dog; and when they take practical steps to do so, encounter bewilderment from those around them who assume they are deluded and crazy. A well-meaning companion tries to explain that there is no dog, that there are no children and that the person with dementia is now a resident in a care home. This information merely has the effect of turning the album back to today's page, leaving them trapped once more in the otherwise insoluble negative ribboning effect which they have been seeking to address – they are now in a state of cruel distress.

Distraction, in the form of a cup of tea, or a short walk, or even a sedative, will not remove the red blanks that have recently been stored. Every time the person catches sight of the negative ribboning effect on today's page they attempt to act to fix the problem. As each of their efforts to use old photographs is impeded by well-meaning carers, they will begin to sink into despair.

Still fully capable of reasoning, they try closing their album altogether in order to escape the sea of insupportable red. They find it preferable to restrict themselves to the black of the outside cover than to open it and risk a return to red. They soon give up opening the album at all. With it closed, much of their ability to establish contact with the world around them is lost. They are in an isolated place, brought on unwittingly, not by dementia but by the well-meaning, if inappropriate, interventions of other people who do not understand. The eventual outcome is a state of near vegetation, a sight which is all too familiar to people working in this field.

A recent report revealed that at the point when they start trying to bury the dog or whatever other action is indicated by the old pages in their photograph albums, a high proportion of current persons with dementia in nursing homes are given extremely powerful anti-psychotic drugs to control their 'mad' behaviour. While it is very understandable that these drugs are administered by staff who may feel it necessary to take desperate measures, studies suggest they makes matters considerably worse. If nothing else, the drugs seem to actually precipitate death in a significant proportion of cases. In one study,[7] over a 12-month period placebo pills (i.e., ones with no active ingredient) were given to a group of Alzheimer's patients and anti-psychotic drugs to another, both groups believing they had been given anti-psychotics. Two years later, the placebo group had a 78 per cent survival rate compared with 54.5 per cent for the drugged. After nearly three and a half years the survival rates were even worse: 60 per cent for the placebos versus only 28 per cent for those given anti-psychotics. There are 244,000 people with dementia living in care homes, of whom about 100,000 are being given anti-psychotic drugs. On the basis of the above study, about 24,000 people a year are dying prematurely as a result of these drugs.

[7] www.telegraph.co.uk/news/main.jhtml?xml=/news/2008/04/01/nalzheim101.xml; Ballard, C. et al, 2008, 'A Randomised, Blinded, Placebo-Controlled Trial in Dementia Patients Continuing or Stopping Neuroleptics (The DART-AD Trial)', *PLoS Medicine*, www.plosmedicine.org, Vol 5, Iss 4, e76.

And yet, it need not be so. Penny has proven that there is another way. Let us return to the confrontation between Dolly and Arthur, that I described earlier. Suppose that they had received Penny's help early on in the development of Dolly's dementia. Arthur has learned about the photograph album analogy and the practical methods described in Part Two of this book. What happens now, at supper time?

Arthur asks if Dolly has posted his letter. Dolly checks back in her album, looking for the information she requires. 'Letter? What letter?' She can find nothing about a letter on this morning's page, so she says that she didn't post it because there was none. *This time*, Arthur nods his head, 'Silly me! My mistake! You're quite right!' Dolly looks at him sympathetically. She tells him not to get concerned as we all tend to be absent-minded when we get older. Arthur agrees and they are soon talking about what a fast-moving world it is, compared to their parents' days. Dolly has stories to tell and Arthur is a good listener. Eventually he suggests that they make their way upstairs and they are soon settling down to sleep.

Neither of them is confused. The state of anxious questioning does not arise. The supper conversation is a new experience and whether it enters Dolly's album as a full photograph or as a blank, it will be an acceptable green. Her life will continue as if the blank at breakfast time had never occurred. The bone of contention between them, that had the capacity to create situations where either might erupt into a temper, has vanished. As blanks continue to build up, Arthur learns to avoid challenging Dolly whenever it is apparent to him that she has not stored a piece of information about herself. He stops asking her questions about the recent past and finds new ways of answering any questions that Dolly herself may pose.

She now spends far less of her life drawing red blanks. As the blanking inexorably builds up, Dolly's capacity to enjoy the repetition of old, recycled green actually increases, unlike people without dementia. If the experience is enjoyable, it remains enjoyable, however many times it is recycled for her. Dolly's life has become uncluttered by unnecessary new facts. Any new ones that she does need, signalling a shift from one activity of daily life to another, are conveyed to her in a context that she understands from her pre-dementia past.

Feeling good, but not knowing why, is a quite different proposition from feeling bad and not knowing why. There is no imperative to take action in response to green. Life becomes peaceful for the older person with dementia who is allowed to draw on such a mass of old photographs. In the final stage of the illness, the current page of the photograph album is almost completely devoid of facts. Yet the repetition of successful links between pre-dementia photographs and all activities of daily life can take place on an ever-simplifying and around-the-clock basis. Penny describes this process as SPECALCARE, where 'care' means continuing acceptable recycled experiences.

USING THE PHOTOGRAPH ALBUM ANALOGY TO PROVIDE SPECALCARE

To recapitulate, Penny offers the simple analogy of a photograph album in order to explain the impact of dementia and to suggest how we might respond to it. The aim is to remove any potential for the red-ribbon effect as soon as possible after diagnosis, in order that the person can enjoy lifelong well-being. Although SPECAL cannot halt the progression of the disease and although new experiences will increasingly be stored as feelings-only blanks, SPECAL can phase out any reliance on new facts. While some new facts will still be stored, it is imperative that they are related in some meaningful way to the pre-dementia past. Penny's work shows that, gradually, it is possible to ensure that all new photographs have positive, green feelings attached. The earlier this process starts the better. You need to carry everyone along with you who is involved with the person with dementia in order to develop continual, appropriate and effective care. So long as carers understand the significance of their own actions and reactions, the personality of the person with dementia can survive. In fact, when this does happen, everyone thrives.

SPECALCARE begins by discreetly uncovering as many old photographs as possible before discovering which ones will be most useful. Once key ones have been identified and successfully brought into use, the family can learn easy ways of passing on the necessary skills to other people coming into regular contact with the person.

Take, for example, Nellie. By the time she was 81, she had been known to the mental health services for three years and was well down the blanking route. Her fiercely loyal, military husband, Richard, was using all his organisational skills in order, as he put it, 'to get the Old Girl sorted'. Nellie had, for her entire marriage, worked quietly in the background of Richard's life, helping his career in countless much-appreciated ways. But now Richard was beginning to see Nellie as a poorly performing member of his regiment. He set about supervising Nellie's life in the house and in the garden. He made list after list, to make sure she knew exactly the plan for each new day. He set himself the task of training Nellie, applying common sense to keep her on the right track. But she had dementia, and common sense memory aids didn't work. In the absence of SPECALCARE, Nellie became increasingly unable to cope.

She wandered about the house creating mayhem in everyone's life. Her attention seemed to focus mainly on drawers and cupboards, which she rummaged through and then emptied all over the place. There were ruinous activities in the garden, too, where she would snip off the heads of flowers as she passed, usually just when they were coming into bloom, leaving an unsightly stalk behind. Nellie would then grumble about the garden to Richard, demanding to know why there was so little colour in it these days. Richard repeatedly pointed out that she was hardly helping in that respect, which made Nellie quite cross and upset. In the little vegetable patch she wrought further havoc, pulling up seedling plants, just as they struggled into life. Richard complained there were no vegetables growing. Nellie had no idea why this could be. Frustration was increasing on both sides and the garden was looking distinctly ill-kempt.

Richard had noticed that Nellie always walked around with a pair of secateurs in her hand, so he had tried hiding them. He reasoned to himself that, 'the poor Old Girl' was 'so far gone these days' that she would soon forget what she was looking for; then the garden would have a chance to recover and Nellie would grumble less. Perhaps, at last, life for them both would improve. But the absence of secateurs completely threw Nellie. She hunted fruitlessly high and low and, as she did so, her sense of confusion grew. Soon she was hunting without knowing what she was hunting for. She looked in every cupboard and drawer in the kitchen, and then moved on upstairs to the bedroom. She grabbed all her clothes out of the cupboard, heaping them up frantically on the bed. She even tried to go up to the attic one day to search there. She could not have said what she was searching for but she was searching for something. The next week she found the door to the attic bolted. Nellie wanted to know why there was a door in the house that she could not open.

This had never happened before. Richard explained over and over again that Nellie's capacity to turn the house upside down was quite intolerable. Nellie, formerly such a placid, gentle and serene lady, became distracted and angry. Richard repeated to the Old Girl for the umpteenth time that there was nothing of interest up there at all, apart from cobwebs and a few bits of worn-out luggage from way back in their old army days.

This was Nellie, then, with all her blanks and a burgeoning collection of reds.

When Penny was consulted, the first step was to get inside Nellie's album. Who was she now, as a person? Who was she before the onset of dementia? Richard was persuaded to turn the pages in his own album back, to tell Penny about how they had met, about Nellie's family, the place where Nellie grew up, their early army experiences together. Who would Nellie have been nowadays, given her age and her life experiences, regardless of dementia? A powerful description emerged. She had been a very keen gardener, as well as a talented flower arranger. Photographs of pruning were everywhere in Nellie's album. They covered a multitude of associated activities, from weeding to dead-heading to picking flowers for arranging in the house, quite apart from the regular autumn clear-up and harvesting vegetables, which led on to cooking, laying the table and other activities that were well-embedded in her memory and featured strongly in her album over many, many years.

All Nellie needed was information from the past to help her in the present. A few simple references, tactfully and subtly supplied, would keep her on track in ways that could become acceptable to everyone. The problem was to convince Richard to replace common sense with SPECALSENSE. He was far from sure that if he changed his attitude, Nellie's old personality would return.

Eventually, and somewhat reluctantly, he went along with the idea of collecting up a large assortment of secateurs and old scissors, broken or otherwise. These were then placed strategically around the house. Secateurs began to appear in many different places, including even the bathroom, which challenged Richard's methodical and disciplined personality. But from Nellie's point of view, wherever she looked, she was almost bound to spot a pair of really useful secateurs. No more risk of drawing a blank. Wandering through the house, her mornings became absorbed in an activity Penny explained to Richard as 'pruning, SPECAL-style', as she moved from one pair of cutters to the next, changing her mind from moment to moment about which pair she might, eventually, use. In between selecting them, she was happy to stop for a cup of coffee with Richard. As that interlude came to an end, she would catch sight of another pair and would return to deciding which to select. Frequently she had still not got round to entering the garden itself before it was time for lunch. Richard soon found that a few minutes spent before the meal deciding where the secateurs ought to be kept safely while she ate made Nellie far more relaxed and conversational throughout the meal.

Another emerging theme from Nellie's old pages related to her health. She had suffered from a minor back problem for years. This had never become a serious ailment and could usually be improved with rest. There were plenty of photographs relating to all this in Nellie's old pages and it became a useful theme to use in her SPECALCARE. Whenever Nellie got as far as the garden, having finally selected her secateurs, Richard would wander up, carrying a lightweight folding chair that he now, after some persuasion, kept in the hall. He also carried a pair of secateurs. Nellie greeted him as a fellow member of the pruning club, suggesting that she give him some handy tips. Richard politely accepted Nellie's guidance as she went about her pruning activities, which were unusual, to say the least. However, Nellie was happy in her role as a competent gardener who was helping someone less expert than herself and, in due course, Richard was able to make a suggestion of his own. He pointed out, quite firmly, that she really ought to rest her back for a while to be sure of remaining fit for what was known in the family as 'the great autumn clear-up'. Richard's language and his tone were familiar to Nellie and resonated with green photographs safely stored in her album many years ago. She was happy to oblige. Now she would sit as he worked, with her secateurs on her lap. She offered her own bits of advice from time to time and was soon chatting about her past achievements in the garden, and elsewhere. Richard didn't get a huge amount of work done in the garden each day but the quality of life for both of them had begun to improve.

By now Richard was becoming confident to act in a SPECAL-informed way and was less insistent about applying common sense. Gardening was a part of Nellie's life again and her morale lifted. She chatted more, throwing light on other information from earlier in her album. Penny learned that she had moved house 23 times during her marriage. Packing and unpacking had been integral to her life. Richard was prevailed upon to take his courage in both hands and unlock the attic. Nellie led Penny up. They peered through the cobwebs as Nellie headed for some luggage stacked in an obscure corner. Under her close instruction, Richard carried an old army trunk downstairs and into the bedroom. The trunk took up a good deal of room and caused Richard some inconvenience but Nellie's life now took another turn for the better. No more piles of clothes left on the bed with nowhere to go. Everything came out of the wardrobe, of course, because Nellie was preparing to move house when she wasn't pruning. Now, indoors as well as out, Nellie knew just what she was up to. In the bedroom, clothes were neatly folded in piles and placed in the trunk ready for the move. When there were rather more clothes in the trunk than in the wardrobe, Nellie went into a magical reverse. Everything was carefully unpacked and put away in the wardrobe. It had become moving-in time. Richard slowly came to recognise that whether Nellie was packing or unpacking was increasingly irrelevant. What mattered was how Nellie felt about it all and she was beginning to feel great. The result was that Richard's morale improved dramatically too. The Old Girl was back on form.

In time, each member of the family developed their own caring techniques when with Nellie but the underlying principles were always the same. Nellie was in touch with intact photographs from the past that were associated with well-being and held her safely in activities that she found very pleasant and, importantly, made sense. These activities in turn triggered further feelings of well-being, which were stored as green. It ceased to be relevant to anyone whether or not the new photographs going into the album were dementia photographs, as long as they were green. Richard was now attaching more importance to Nellie's feelings than to the facts of what she was doing. 'Moving house' and 'pruning' entered the family vocabulary as meaningful phrases for Nellie, as each day she gently oscillated between the two. It became relatively easy to connote these activities by a few familiar gestures.

SPECALCARE was narrowing the gap between who Nellie had been and who Nellie was now. The emerging profile of a day in her life was beginning to look like the sort of day that she had always enjoyed. She felt herself to be back in her previously well-established role and in control of her life once more.

Still more information from Nellie's album emerged. This time it concerned Nellie's view of sailing, and more specifically, Richard's boat. Richard had named the boat Nell, after Nellie, but it was affectionately known in the family as 'the bloody boat'. The words tripped from Nellie's lips in a delightfully light way. Nellie had always suffered from seasickness, which meant she was thrilled to be excused any visit to Nell, provided she didn't feel that she was letting Richard down. Common sense suggested referring to the boat only when Richard was actually going sailing. But SPECALSENSE made use of nautical prompts to explain any absence by Richard, *whether or not he was physically on board his boat at the time*. Whenever a family member or friend provided Nellie with a murmured reference to sailing if Richard was out of sight, she would respond with a smile, saying, 'Oh, the bloody boat! I'm glad I've been let off!' With that she would happily settle into her task of preparing for their next house move.

The disease progressed and Nellie's cognitive function continued to decline but her sense of well-being remained firmly in place. Much of the detail of Nellie's personalised themes gradually reduced over time as the dementia ticked on. By now, a simple gesture of a rocking hand became sufficient to convey the idea of 'the bloody boat' to Nellie. In due course she moved smoothly into a nursing home and carried on her life's routines there, hardly noticing the move. The connections between the past and the present continued to work, and the essence of her life was retained to the end. The trunk eventually evolved into a small handbag that accompanied her wherever she went. Several hankies were packed and unpacked; even a small piece of paper on Nellie's bedroom chair provided something for her to fold.

Richard visited Nellie each week in the nursing home. He described her state of mind as 'serene'. They sat and chatted together, each in their own way. Nellie's back slowly improved – or so she said, politely, if anyone enquired. She would explain that the packing was going quite well, too. She was content that Richard was involved with 'the bloody boat' whenever he was missing. Each day was familiar and comforting and only after a good many years did the day in the life of Nellie come full circle as she packed her handbag for the last time.

And Richard? Where does all this leave Richard? At the suggestion of SPECAL his time is increasingly taken up with a new interest that gradually spread into his life as Nellie's dependence on him grew less. He chose marine history, and this has been a lifeline to him. He has sold his boat and spends his time on a newly acquired computer, writing a book for the family about his own sailing history. He misses Nellie very much but tells everyone that he also achieves a feeling of contentment each day as he reflects on how he managed to make, for Nellie, a present of the past.

Nellie's story illustrates how the analogy of the photograph album informs SPECALCARE. With this understanding in place, you are ready to learn the practical techniques.

Part Two

HOW TO PROVIDE 24-HOUR WRAPAROUND CARE

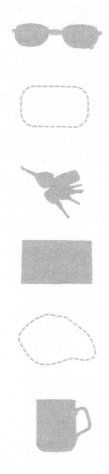

Introduction

With Part One under your belt, you are ready to learn the SPECAL method for delivering 24-hour wraparound care for lifelong well-being.

From this point on, although it may seem a bit weird at first, I shall refer to the person with dementia as your 'client'. If that person is your close relative, this is particularly likely to seem uncomfortably impersonal, but as you will see in Parts Two and Three, you are going to be asked to take a very professional approach and to acquire new skills. Part of the crucial shift now needed is to think of the person with dementia as somebody who is your client.

To briefly recap, the SPECAL method is designed to achieve two fundamental goals:

1. Protection from having to store new information:
This is achieved by creating a social environment in which the client is never required to try and recall something from the recent past. Everyone whom the client meets is prepared in

such a way that it does not matter that information on recent pages has not been stored.

2. Support through old photographs when new information is required:
In the absence of more recent information, people with dementia are liable to interpret what is happening around them as being a situation from the past. The SPECAL technique turns this natural tendency to consult old pages in their album – which common sense would stigmatise as 'confusing the past with the present' – into a salvation. It enables clients to live contentedly in the present through the past.

To achieve the first goal of never challenging clients with new information, carers must learn to replace common sense with SPECALSENSE, based on three commandments:

- Don't ask questions.
- Learn from them as the experts on their disability.
- Always agree with everything they say, never interrupting them.

Chapters 4–6 teach you how to follow these injunctions and provide three new ways of communicating and understanding. The first is to converse with clients using 'verbal ping-pong' (Chapter 4). The second is to spot the most commonly asked questions that your client keeps repeating and to identify acceptable answers to them (Chapter 5). And the third is to employ conversational loops for getting the client from red to green (Chapter 6).

Just obeying the three commandments will, in itself, reap rapid rewards. Implementing the new skills will do the same. Not only will the client quickly become much less confused and irritable, you will be able to communicate infinitely better with them, heralding a much better state of mind for yourself. You will now be ready to achieve the second goal: the creation of a system for ensuring that old photographs are being used in the most effective manner, explained in Chapters 7–9.

First, you have to identify the client's Primary Theme (Chapter 7). This is a narrative from the client's past that is going to underpin much of their waking life. It will provide them with a continuing sense of achievement gained from a particular area of past expertise, no matter how modest. The narrative may concern having been a traveller, baker, munitions factory manager, lollipop lady, whatever. More than anything else, it is this Primary Theme which enables the method to work over a 24-hour cycle and makes it wraparound, in the sense that it can operate at all times and in all places, a true safety blanket against new information.

Second, you have to identify a Health Theme (Chapter 8). The Primary Theme is so powerful in its promotion of independence that a balancing mechanism is required to reconnect the client to their need for help in essential everyday life activities, like eating, sleeping and managing continence. The Health Theme does this job; a medical topic from the client's past, like a recurring back problem or old operation on their knee. It's something they would acknowledge has caused them to rely on other people to help out for a while, and they can do so with dignity and without getting depressed. Yes, they may still be a traveller waiting for their plane or a manager organising their munitions factory, but they can accept that they have a reason (nothing to do with dementia) to accept help from other people, so they agree they need to get some sleep or have something to eat or spend time in the bathroom, in between their expert activities.

Third, you have to identify acceptable Explanations for who is present or absent in the client's social environment (Chapter 9). The reasons given need to be stored on the client's old pages, they will be no help if they have had to be memorised as new data. Clients can easily become alarmed because they lack useful information about who is who, what they are doing and why. They are also concerned with where key figures in their life may have gone. As the main carer, you need an acceptable explanation for why you have to briefly leave the room. You need another one that can be used by someone else to explain your absence if you are gone for several hours. And you need a third explanation for why that someone else is there. How is the client to know the difference between a complete stranger – a robber, perhaps – and someone they are happy to accept in their house?

Once you have absorbed all this and put it into practice, you are providing 24-hour wraparound care that sustains lifelong well-being. However, there are two further practical steps that are needed before you are completely sorted. The first is that you need to train a team for providing the care. 'Team' is being used here in the loosest possible sense to include absolutely everyone the client comes into contact with. Chapter 11 explains how to do this so that everyone starts relating to the client in ways that rely on old, rather than new information, and no one challenges the safety blanket provided by the Primary Theme (e.g., by saying 'this isn't an airport lounge' or 'this is not a munitions factory').

The final step is to identify the nursing home in which your client is very likely to eventually live. This may seem like a deeply depressing thing to be thinking about at this stage and one best left well alone. However, for reasons explained in Part Three, the family home will at some point become an emotionally challenging place from the client's perspective and they will need the relative peace of a nursing home. This is SPECALSENSE. Common sense makes families feel they must set their sights on being able to ensure that the client remains at home until the end of their life, yet this long-term aim is not in the best interests of the client. Importantly, if the family persists with this aim, they will find themselves in a crisis far earlier than would otherwise have been the case. Also, if you use SPECALCARE it will actually delay the point at which a care home is required. The Royal College of Nursing evaluation found that the SPECAL method, with its early focus on planning an eventual move, has the effect of delaying, not accelerating, a move away from home.

Now that the whole future is laid out before you, you are all set to learn the method. The only other thing you need is a pen and a new notebook – from now on you will need to adopt a daily routine of recording a few observational notes. From time to time I will also ask you to do simple exercises.

Remember, if something is not making sense or you are getting stuck, you can always seek support from www.specal.co.uk, and you may find helpful written material at www.oliver-james-books.com.

CHAPTER FOUR

Don't Ask Questions

The ideas described in the next few paragraphs are almost guaranteed to bring a rapid improvement in the well-being of the client and also of yourself. The remainder of the chapter provides a whole new way of relating to the client that will entrench this advance, to your mutual advantage.

The ostensibly simple advice is to *cease asking your client any direct questions at all and aim never to ask them another one*. Actually, this is easier said than done, and I will provide detailed instructions on how to learn not to ask questions and what to do instead, in a moment. But first, you need to understand why questions are as poisonous to the well-being of people with dementia as radiation is to the health of newborn babies.

Before we get started you might like to get a cup of tea or coffee, to help you concentrate – do you want one? In order to decide your answer, note that you have to ask yourself a series of further questions: 'Have I just had a drink? Do I want to interrupt reading this now? Haven't I given up caffeine drinks? Have we got any milk?' and so on. You have to consult recent pages in your photograph album. Assuming you do not have dementia, you can run through the various issues at lightning speed, quickly finding the relevant photographs to answer your sub-questions (photographs indicating 'given up caffeine', 'just had one', etc.) and perhaps very quickly conclude that you want to get on with reading this section rather than be interrupted.

If I have dementia it is a very different matter. When I consult my album I may find little or almost no information on today's page. Turning further back, I have a collection of damaged pages all the way to where the blanking first began. Fundamentally, although I have had plenty of cups of tea in my life, I may have insufficient numbers of photographs to tell me whether it is appropriate to have a cup of tea right now. Will I be the only person having one? Will the questioner have to go miles to get it? Will I hold everyone up if I say yes? Each one of these internal questions poses a problem to me, one by one. To answer them, I must search the recent pages, which is very liable to distress and confuse me.

To make matters worse I may not even be storing the question in its entirety, so as I try to attend to the follow-on internal stuff I get lost. I am asking myself what I am looking for. Even that information is not properly stored. Help! Within a split second of being asked I am in a maze, beginning to panic. The questioner looks at me slightly strangely and repeats it, very kindly and patiently. The whole process starts again. I am seconds away from becoming very alarmed indeed by new questions that I am about to ask myself, like 'What is the name of the questioner?', 'Where am I?' and then, 'Is there not something very seriously wrong with me indeed if I am having such trouble answering such a simple question?' followed very possibly by, 'What question – have I been asked a question? It seems this person is waiting for an answer, but I don't know what I have been asked.' So, being asked a seemingly simple direct question has caused me potentially catastrophic and largely unseen anguish that wasn't there before.

The toxicity of questions was something Penny Garner learned from observing her mother. On one occasion, Penny and her parents were at lunch with friends when the hostess asked who would like a second helping. That question always puts one slightly on the spot. Issues flash up like 'Is there enough to go round?' and 'If I say yes, will I be the only one?' Penny went through the usual split second 'yes or no' process and decided to decline. She glanced across as her mother was asked and saw her face turn grey. She had always been disarmingly decisive but now she reacted in a most uncharacteristic way. Dorothy glanced at her plate, perhaps wondering whether they had just eaten at all. She looked around at everyone else and back to the hostess. Now she didn't seem to grasp what she was being offered more of. She peered towards Sam as if to say, 'Help! Have we got time? What is everyone else doing? Who is doing what here, exactly?' She seemed totally baffled, clearly in mental anguish.

Penny's heart sank when Sam provided a peremptory prompt: 'Dorothy, do get a move on. You are holding everyone up.' But in response her mother's face cleared and she rose to her feet. 'Come on, Sam. We mustn't hold things up. We've had a lovely time and we really must say goodbye.' She had never suffered from porch paralysis, always the one to thank, turn and leave in a single move. But this time her husband didn't rise with her. Instead, he told her to sit down and the grey face returned, now with a completely defeated look. Until then, no one had thought there was anything wrong with her at all. Suddenly, here was yet another sign that she had a terrible disease that was tragically destroying her ability to join in socially or even, at times, to speak.

Afterwards, pondering what had prompted such a rapid shift from social ease to a near-zombie state, Penny realised it was the question. It demanded information Dorothy did not have about the events that immediately preceded it. That also made sense of the sudden rise from the table to depart. She thought that Sam had provided her with a clue that she must move. She took the context he had offered and acted on it, completely in character. She had not lost her personality, but she was thinking she was at a party from yester-year, long before her illness, not the one they were actually at now. In consulting photograph pages representing lunch parties from long ago, Dorothy had returned to one of these. No wonder she was so poleaxed when told to sit down again. It questioned the whole basis of her reality as profoundly as it would question yours if I was able to prove to you right now that you are someone other than the person whose name is on your birth certificate.

Penny rapidly learned from this incident the difference between direct questions, which demand an answer, and statements or imperatives that merely encourage participation. It became abundantly clear that direct questions were harmful. In their stead, Penny gradually found herself using a range of opening gambits in which the most important word was 'we': 'I wonder if we should . . .', 'It might be a good idea if we . . .'. Dorothy invariably had views if Penny started a sentence like that and they were fairly predictable, based on much-repeated stuff from the past. Dorothy was the person she always had been, so long as she was drawing from the older photographs. As we shall see, the carer needs to become a master at introducing the we-relationship in a deliberately meandering speech style.

Unfortunately, this was not Sam's style. He was keen on facts and getting them right made him feel good. The lunch saga unfolded every time they were asked out. He used to regale Penny with the same story; different people, different venues, but always the same outcome. In Sam's view, Dorothy had been embarrassing to all concerned and socially unacceptable. However hard Penny tried to explain where the problem was coming from, she never made progress with him. He would exclaim, 'I really don't see at all what you're talking about Penny! You seem to have lost all grip on common sense.'

When Penny was present she could firefight in advance. She had to remain extremely vigilant to get in quick to provide information that would subsume any question asked, and it worked. Her mother was as if there was nothing wrong with her at all. But if Penny wasn't there the occasion was almost invariably catastrophic. Her father would keep Dorothy 'up to the mark', getting more and more nervous that she would let him down, and his feelings of anxiety transferred to her. She had no idea what he was anxious about, but it made her anxious too.

Knowing the toxicity of questions, when first working at Burford Penny watched with horror as clients were put through their paces from the moment they walked through the door: 'Did you have a good journey?', 'Is it raining outside?', 'How is this . . . how is that . . . did you this . . . did you that . . .', the normal language of common sense. She began to see patterns in how they coped with it. They either froze while they went through the 'Now let me think' bit, or they answered the question off the top of their head without thinking at all. The latter was fascinating to observe. She heard a client answer a question about what they had done yesterday in a variety of ways, from 'It was pouring with rain so I stayed in and polished the brass' to 'It was hot and sunny and I went to Weston-Super-Mare with the family' – different each time. The hospital care assistant saw the clients' answers as evidence that they were making things up, whereas to Penny it was obvious they were using information from old pages in their albums. There was no photograph available of what precisely had happened the day before, so they consulted pages from weeks or years before with relevant weather information and general news, happening upon a different page each time, so providing different answers. They had not lost their reason, far from it, but they were clearly drastically short of recent information. The care assistant became less and less interested in what she saw as meaningless conversation going nowhere, and merely recorded 'confused' in the notes at the end of the day. Penny found herself wondering who the notes were about – the patient or the staff.

The whole hospital system, whether in the Day Unit or hospital inpatient departments, was based on an 'assessment of need' that required questions. Assessment prior to a rehabilitation programme is common sense and Burford's reputation for rehabilitation was second to none. However, once you understand what is wrong with people with dementia it is horrifying to realise that the main method for establishing how the person can be helped is itself a major cause of emotional distress. As a way of driving them crazy, it was, unwittingly, highly effective. Questions, questions, questions. It is common sense to ask them but it did not work for the SPECAL clients. They already had a diagnosis of an irreversible condition and were ready for rehabilitation of a very specialised and different sort.

Luckily, Burford Hospital turned out to be ideal as a clinical laboratory for exploring alternatives that fitted with SPECALSENSE. In the early days the nurses asked Penny to find out the answers to what they felt they needed to know because the process took quite a bit of time – far more than with a non-SPECAL patient. However, in the long run it saved so much time and so minimised stress that the staff began incorporating the technique into their routines. No questions = happy, well-functioning client. Questions = eventual havoc as the stress and strain gradually built up to boiling point, usually at the end of the day. Almost all problems with clients turned out to have been caused by the staff applying common sense, and questioning was a prime suspect on each occasion.

Indeed, the very process of arriving at red has its origins in questions. Even if everyone avoids asking the client a direct question, the client is bound to be asking themselves questions (mostly silently) for much of the time. When they first start questioning, they are unlikely to be anywhere near red (deep trauma) – they are a long way off – but the point is that they are moving in that direction. They are, as it were, on amber. Amber is a signal to alert the carer, a warning sign: the client needs information and is starting a search. There is, at this point, the potential for them either to head back to the safety of green, or to slide insidiously and ultimately catastrophically towards a new red blank in the present. What the client needs, all the time, is help in reaching old intact pages of their album so that they can get useful green photographs at speed. The substitute information they need, and must be offered, is just as useful to them as a pair of artificial legs to an amputee. Left alone to leaf back on amber, they will be asking themselves more and more unanswerable questions, and end up on hideous red.

To understand this better, before you begin doing anything directly with the client, you need to practise on someone else – someone without dementia. The following exercise will help.

> **EXERCISE: Not asking questions**
>
> The next time you are having a 15-minute chat with someone without dementia, try to get through your entire conversation without asking them any questions at all. You will quickly see how hard it is. Notice the strategies you employ as alternatives. For example, instead of asking if your conversational partner would like a cup of tea directly, you may turn it around and state, 'I think I will have a cup of tea', and by nonverbal means, like a shrug or a look, encourage the person to volunteer for one. This can be built upon by using the inclusive 'we', and by giving statements such as 'maybe it's time for us to have a cup of tea' a rhetorical, questioning air, through a raised pitch at the end of the sentence, without requiring answers.

Once you have practised on someone without dementia, you can give it a go with the client, and if you really do avoid questions, you will immediately notice how much more forthcoming they become. However, avoiding questions is not in itself enough. Now that you are becoming expert at avoiding questions yourself you are ready for a whole new way of communicating with the client.

VERBAL PING-PONG

Most carers find it becomes increasingly hard to have enjoyable conversations with the client. Casual chatting breaks down quickly as the client seems to lose track of the subject, or to change it randomly. The fluent to-and-fro exchange of news and views becomes elusive and in its absence, both feel isolated, lonely. It's an important part of normal intimacy and the dispirited carer's consequent negative mood makes the client anxious. A dark spiral of silence develops, inter-rupted only by dreary and frustratingly repetitive questions from the client eliciting similarly tinged answers, ones that are increasingly not stored by the client, leading to yet further repetition of their question.

Penny's phrase for the technique which breaks out of this gruesome pattern is 'verbal ping-pong'. By this, she does not mean the usual cut and thrust, in which you do all in your power to win. In this version, only the client wins or at best, there's an honourable draw. That doesn't sound much like fun, but as you will see, once you have learned to play in this counter-intuitive fashion it will vastly refresh your relationship with the client and thereby improve their well-being. Not only that, it is a very important means by which you will be able to involve other people in caring for the client, to give you the breaks that are essential if you are to keep going yourself. The skill you are about to acquire is one that can be easily taught to a stranger who has never met the client – one that they will be able to enjoy together for hours on end.

Before starting, you need to think about all the client's favourite subjects of conversation, things that are of real interest or concern to them. The topics could be anything at all and might well be something that they no longer do, like an old hobby or sport. Think of their favourite stories reflecting confidence and well-being. See what you can come up with as you try out the following exercise.

EXERCISE: Your client's favourite topic

In your notebook write down *your client's* favourite words or phrases. Try to think of this exercise as an amusing game rather than a chore. Do not worry, plenty of ideas will come to mind.

Identify three topics from the words or phrases that you think may trigger a familiar patter (however brief) from the client.

These topics are the verbal ping-pong balls that you will use. They should always reflect the client's past interests rather than any of your own. Having selected these balls as potential sources of conversation, you are ready to start playing, with one proviso: only try it out at first for very short periods. It is hard work to start with and you need to focus exclusively on the game. Better by far to clear the decks of any distraction and spend a short time, say 10 minutes of quality play, when you are not half listening out for the phone or wondering if the potatoes are boiling over. You need your full attention on the client and the game, so at first, don't overdo it.

Just as you might try a certain amount of tapping the ball up and down on your bat, or flicking of the bat to try out a few shots, you start with a few limbering comments. At this point you are not even hitting a ball (favourite topic) over the net; so far there are no points to score, you're not even knocking up. What you do is to burble and babble in a manner you never usually would. You might say, 'Well, gosh, I don't know' or 'Hmm, this weather never seems to change' or 'Here we go then, now then, hum, I don't know', talking about nothing at all really, just burble burble burble, totally unthreatening, not in the slightest way trying to engage the person directly in conversation. It will not be at all like the way you normally converse, you are just waffling about neutral generalities: 'Good lord, it looks like autumn out there', 'It's nice and warm in here', 'Glad I wrapped up warm this morning.' The knock-up at your end is so inconsequential and unchallenging that the client will not have to 'think' about what you are saying in any serious way. What you are doing is getting alongside them, moving into their orbit, onto their radar, as you become a vaguely benign component in their immediate emotional force-field.

After a bit of this, you can begin to start knocking the occasional ball over the net in their general direction without aiming it directly at them. You see if they pick it up and if not, you are ready with another ball to lob casually over the net. The absolute key from now on is that, through the topic you have chosen, you are looking for them to engage, to pick it up, to return it, and at that point you can stay with that topic and lob another gentle response back to them. You are inwardly alert, on your toes, spotting moments when they become alive, involved and engaging in the rally, without really noticing that it has started. You are always playing from the position that they are the expert, the teacher, and you are the pupil. You will be the one with the less-than-perfect memory, from time to time throwing in the odd shot of 'Now, let me see, I'm not sure I remember what exactly happened that day.' You take the position of someone who is happy to be instructed by the other player. You are deliberately going to seek out areas in which the client feels themselves to be competent, based on the photographs in the early pages in their album, and you are going to give them opportunities to tell you all about what you cannot precisely remember but would like to know. Hence, if one of their interests is baking cakes, you might start with 'Cakes sometimes rise but not always. I wonder about cakes, I really do.' Varying your words very slightly each time increases your chances of picking up their interest. At first you would be speaking to yourself, making no attempt to direct the comment at them, just burbling. If there is no response, you need not worry. Let the dementia work for you: if you repeat the subject in a few seconds' time, they will almost certainly have failed to store your first effort.

If by any chance they point out that you are getting extraordinarily repetitive (highly unlikely but never to be ruled out), you immediately play one of the most useful shots in your repertoire – it is called 'Silly me! You're right! Goodness me!' Don't look on this as a failure. There's no such thing as right or wrong in verbal ping-pong, just what works for the other player, and you will only know that when they return the ball. 'Silly me, the carer' is a vast improvement on 'Silly you, the client' as you will already be finding out. The 'Silly me' return will do for anything where the client is querying what you are saying.

When you spot a word or phrase or comment that engages the client, you can try repeating it. This time allow your eye to look towards them and your body language to show that you are including them in your musing, by turning in their direction. In doing so, you are offering them a gentle lob that they can decide whether or not to hit back. If they want to bash it out of court, fine – never disagree with their choice of shot. If it's of no interest they will let it go past them, that's not a problem either, merely a signal that the rally is not under way, so you pause politely and try a different ball. Whereas in the normal ping-pong of conversation you are hoping to score points and prefer to serve aces, the opposite is the case here, you want the client to do so. Rather than serve the ball away from the opponent so they cannot return it, in this version you want it to go smack bang to the very (psychological) place where they are.

The moment they hit something back you must lock on to it, whatever it is. However peculiar, apparently unrelated to your opening topic, always go with it. A rally is beginning. Now, inwardly, you are going to have to become very active and downright clever, using all your imagination, although outwardly what you say and do may often seem banal. Once the game has started, you really will have to perform, to be an actor, and yet at all times you will also be working hard to be as authentic as you possibly can. On reading those words you may be thinking, 'Oh God, don't expect me to be amusing or clever or diverting. Right now it's the last thing I feel.' But do not worry. You will be rewarded so rapidly by their response that you will feel tremendously encouraged, lifting you up and giving you the pleasure of feeling connected to the person.

You want to start identifying the highly idiosyncratic ways in which they reveal that they enjoy a topic, when a rally seems to be beginning. It is easy to spot when they become chatty, animated and engaged but that is unlikely to occur immediately. They may have particular looks that precede engagement, perhaps a sideways glance to check you are with them. They may have specific hand gestures, a raised finger to attract attention. Their body might alter its position, so that they raise their shoulders and look you in the eye. The more expert you become at identifying such patterns, the easier it will become to get them engaged in a rally.

In responding, try to match and mirror their language and body movements. The more self-aware and alert you are, the better your performance. Perhaps they speak very slowly and deliberately – then do so too, likewise if they are speedy. Listen out for specific turns of phrase and be ready to feed that particular combination of words back to them a bit later, to make them feel they are among friends. Perhaps during a rally about dogs, the client refers positively to someone as being 'a bit of a shaggy one', then you could refer a minute later to a mutual acquaintance as being 'another shaggy one' or try turning the phrase into 'we', making yourselves the shaggy ones – yes, I really am suggesting that you be as self-consciously steering of events as this. Even directly mirror the rhythm of their words so that if they say a word like 'daffodil', you might say something like 'daffodil . . . on the hill . . .' while planning your next shot. You could muse on about daffodils being golden because that way you're getting close to a golden retriever dog and back to shaggy ones, if that's the ball that seems to work best.

Once you have tried it you will soon see that there are endless possibilities for finding ways of gently nudging conversations. The client will have no problem with apparently nonsensical statements from time to time so long as it feels like a really pleasant, non-threatening fireside chat.

At every opportunity they must be aware that what they are saying is working very well on the feelings level. Think feelings, not facts. Do not be afraid to actually say things that you have never, until this moment, ever felt about the subject, like 'how interesting', 'wow, I'm learning something new here', 'gosh, who would have thought that'. Liberal flattery and total fascination greatly help them to feel the game is pleasurable. They badly need reassurance of their own personal worth, something that has been slipping away from them since the diagnosis. It may feel insincere to say things you do not feel or believe but at a deeper level you are trying to improve their well-being. If you can only begin to restore this, you will be restoring some of your own sanity and quality of life as well.

Constantly encourage the idea that you two are engaged in a conspiratorial alliance: that 'we' are doing something together; that everyone else is outside. If a third person appears, give that person a meaningful look to convey the idea that something important is going on between you and the client. If interrupted, you might say 'Thank you, we're just discussing shaggy dogs', giving the client a knowing, 'I'm your best friend' look. The game takes precedence over every other social nicety involving other people. The game is for two; you and your best friend, the client. You cannot afford for the ball to be missed, you have to sustain the conversation because it is the place where the client is safe. It is important to realise that however much you may offend a spectator on the sidelines of the game, that is a better situation by far than risking the emotional safety of the client, which is being protected by the rally they are currently engaging in with you. People without dementia can recover from small dents to their self-esteem and you can explain this to them at some other time. There is no such luxury when it comes to client care. The client is more vulnerable, more important, than any spectator. It is as simple as that.

You will know the game is completely underway when it begins to take longer and longer for the ball to come back. They have taken to bouncing it up and down on their own racquet, chatting away as part of the process of sending it back. When it eventually arrives on your side of the net, it will take only a tap to get it back to them, maybe just a nod or a mutually resonant word, then they will be happily off again. Once absorbed, playing with a ball they delight in, they are no longer questioning, they are totally engaged in describing or discussing or debating whatever is on the table. However, just because they seem to be well away, you must not fall asleep. Your intimate eye-contact, your nods and smiles, these all have a crucial part to play. You have to stay inwardly alert, thinking ahead and observing them closely because it is always up to you to ensure they remain safely in this place where no new information is liable to burst in and upset their fragile coracle of well-being.

Once you have learned to play this game, you will have found one or more topics that are guaranteed to light up the client. You will also have a few key words which trigger interest in each topic and you will have a good feel for how to keep the ball in play for longer periods. Be sure to note it down in your book because, as a carer, you are a busy, stretched person and may need to remind yourself of the details of what works. This information is gold dust because you can impart it easily to other carers and soon you will be able to involve all sorts of other people in ping-pong with the client while you, seamlessly, are able to leave them to it and have time out for yourself.

EXERCISE: Your favourite topic

Forget the world of dementia just for a moment, and select an area of particular and enduring interest from your own life that you would be happy to chat with someone about at length. In my case it would be 'dribbling' (as in footballs, rather than saliva – I was quite a dab hand with my feet).

Imagine you have been introduced to someone new who seems pleasant and friendly. You soon discover that they have always been fascinated by this subject, although they do not appear to be particularly expert. Now ask yourself what question they could ask you which would be of maximum interest to answer (my abiding issue was always, 'How does one best blend dribbling with team play?').

If you imagine yourself answering this question, what themes might emerge in it? (For me it would be things like, George Best versus Maradona, selfishness versus selflessness.)

Now let's return to the world of dementia. If you stop to think about it, you can probably see that if you had dementia and someone started talking about your chosen topic, so long as they seemed genuinely interested and well disposed, you would soon be chatting away. If, furthermore, they had worked out in advance that certain questions were of particular fascination to you and raised them in rhetorical form (e.g., speaking to me, it might be 'I suppose it must always be a big problem deciding the best moment to pass', which could set me off for hours), you can see that you might happily bore for Britain on this topic. So if your conversationalist took careful note of the themes that arose during your answers, you can also see that they could be raised again and again during future conversations on the topic.

> Given that you have dementia, repetition would not be a problem because you would not have stored the fact of having already covered this subject in this way.

Applied to your client, you can also see how helpful this technique could be. If you can get them on to their favourite topic, finding the right triggers for activating their interest in it, you can also recycle the themes they develop, introducing them whenever the conversation seems to be lagging. The person with dementia is insulated from boredom with what they enjoy in a way that you and I without dementia can only admire. Familiarity does not breed contempt, repetition becomes an absolute boon.

TROUBLESHOOTING

Here are some of the main difficulties encountered by carers when embarking on verbal ping-pong.

'I refuse to even try the game because it's deceitful, isn't it?'

The commonest objection felt by carers before even starting to play is that ping-pong is 'manipulative', 'deceitful' or 'lying'. If you are a spouse or partner, you may feel that it is uncomfortable to so cold-bloodedly (as it may seem) and deliberately fashion a discussion topic, to pretend to find the answers interesting, to pre-plan issues and themes for further prompting. You may also find it distressing. Here was someone with whom you shared your life, who may have been a formidable intellect or was a canny mover and shaker, yet now your conversation is reduced to this seemingly empty charade, in which your responses are confected and false. If you are an offspring, you may find it heart-rending to have to 'spoon-feed' a once powerful, impressive parent with little smatterings of their favourite hobby-horses. Whatever your relationship, you may also find it exhausting and a step too far to have to boost their esteem with a constant flow of insincere compliments and encouragement, pretending to find what they say fascinating when in fact, its repetitiousness and predictability fills you with a mixture of boredom and frustration, as well as a sadness that this wonderful person has been reduced to such a 'pathetic' level. You may feel that if anyone needs boosting, it's you. Your morale may be low because you almost feel as if you have suffered a bereavement, as if the loved one you once knew has died. You may feel that despite massive quantities of (probably wholly unacknowledged by anyone) time and energy poured into caring for the client, you are failing them, because they seem so confused and unhappy. That lowers your self-esteem, so it's you who needs to feel valued, not them.

That you feel any, or all, of these things is wholly understandable. However, you will rapidly cease to think like this the moment you get some rallies with the client going.

Firstly, you will see that you are wholly authentic in your dealing with the client, despite the fact that you are sometimes simulating interest and are manufacturing the subject matter more than you would usually do (for, of course, all of us must necessarily sometimes lead conversations in normal life in the directions that we want them to go; as T.S. Eliot put it, in order to join normal social exchanges you must 'put on a face to meet the faces that you meet'). Because you understand the limitations that dementia places on the client's information storage, you are crafting the conversation for their benefit. But it's much more than that. As well as revitalising your interactions with the client through ping-pong and the techniques to be explained in succeeding chapters, you are going to make all the difference in the world to the client's well-being.

If you go back to the exercise and imagine you really have got dementia, would you not want your carer to find a topic about which you can talk, and to feed you helpful tips, providing the external scaffolding which you no longer possess internally? Would you not want them to boost you so you have the confidence to keep on conversing? Would you not want them to start every interaction on the basis that you can no longer store new facts? Of course you would, and this gives you, as the carer, the consent you need to help them in the way proposed.

Another basic problem is that you may be feeling so low (exhausted, undermined, overwhelmed) that the idea of trying verbal ping-pong just seems too much. Again, I have to tell you that playing the game is truly the only way out of this state of mind; you have just got to try it. I realise that some readers will feel this sounds like the spurious snakeoil of positive psychology self-help. But at least as important as what the game will achieve for the client is the help it will give you. Once you have got the hang of it you will feel a million times less lonely, a flood of relief that the person you knew is still there, that you can express and receive affection with them. You will also feel massively more able to believe that you can handle this thing, that it is *not* an impenetrable, hopeless downhill struggle whose only resolution can be the client's death or their incarceration in a nursing home.

'What if I don't do trivial small talk?'

You may be someone who has never been any good at small talk, so the burbling, babbling initial stage may seem completely at variance with your normal style. You may also be a man – a lot of men say they can't abide chitchat, that they only enjoy conversation about really important or serious matters.

Bob used to be like this. He was someone who 'always ends up helping out with the washing up or passing round the crisps at parties' because he simply could not think what to say if someone's opening gambit was that the weather has been nice or that they had a traffic-free journey to the party. Unless he found a person who wanted to get into a heavy, intense discussion concerning something about which he was well informed, he did not enjoy socialising.

For such people, pretence and game-playing often do not come naturally. The answer is, however, that this is not about the normal small talk or tittle-tattle or trivia of everyday conversation, this is a situation which requires the carer to engage all their wits in the service of their loved one and themselves. Once they grasp this, in most cases the problem goes away. Almost anyone can perform the role of someone who is slightly confused and uncertain, necessary to the initial stages of the game. If they think consciously of themselves as engaging in a role play, it becomes much easier. Penny has often said that the best training for a SPECAL carer is some time spent at acting school. By planning in advance what the carer's burbling will be – 'Oh dear, there never seems to be enough time', 'Gosh, the traffic is so bad' or whatever – they can take away the problem. They just need to learn their lines and act the part. In having to be proactive and targeted, they quickly realise this is interesting and important. It is a vital exercise in trying to foster communication with a loved one who lacks the capacity to store new information, a challenging, interesting problem, not idle chinwagging.

When Bob became a SPECAL carer he had real difficulties with verbal ping-pong but he soon discovered for himself that it was worth the effort to change his approach: 'I found it almost impossible at first but now I could talk the hind legs off a donkey,' he says today, 'and it's enabled me to get my wife back.'

'What do I do if the client suspects I am being patronising?'

From time to time, even experienced players will hit the ball too hard or in the wrong place, risking an end to the whole game. The client may begin to tire of the subject but most commonly, what sends them to amber is when the carer says something which suddenly makes the client question what is going on.

For example, Penny was able to play many hours of ping-pong with her mother Dorothy using the ball of air travel. On one occasion, Penny had allowed her attention to wander as Dorothy chatted through one of her favourite stories. Penny realised with a jolt that it was her shot, that Dorothy was waiting for a response, and she knocked a ball carelessly back over the net to her mother with the ill-chosen words 'Gosh, I had no idea you are allowed so much hand luggage on flights.' Dorothy immediately raised her eyebrows and gave her a penetrating look, one that spoke louder than words. Penny knew it meant, 'but you know perfectly well that lots of luggage is permitted'. She knew that her mother could rapidly move on to thinking 'Is Penny stringing me along in some way? And if so, why? Am I not making sense here?'

All clients store some facts at all stages of the illness and it's impossible to guess in advance when it will happen. While the pretence and simulation entailed in ping-pong will be invisible for the vast majority of the time, occasionally the illusory nature of what is happening (however much it is an illusion based on an authentic reality) can suddenly seem exposed.

An interesting parallel is what can happen when playing fantasy games with children around the age of five. I used to play a game with my daughter on the beach searching for pirate treasure in the sand. She would ask me to suggest good places to look and, lo and behold, individual coins would appear. When we first played, there was no sign that she realised I was sneaking the coins into the sand. However, from the age of three onwards, in playing other fantasy games she did enjoy occasionally blowing the gaffe and exposing the greasepaint, suddenly saying, 'You're not a real monster, Dada, you're Dada', either because the game was getting too scary or too boring. Heading for the beach aged five, she mused, 'Dada, it's strange that I only find treasure in the sand when I search with you.' Sure enough, she soon caught me red-handed planting a coin. Interestingly, however, this did not lead to recrimination or any sign that she felt she had been swizzed. On the contrary, she says she is looking forward to the hunt next year. This indicates that from a young age we can share a pretence without feeling defrauded by each other.

In all interactions we frequently employ an 'as if' mode, so that I might put on a funny voice to entertain a friend or speak of myself with irony, and they will know that I am still me. However, for the parallel with my daughter to apply to the occasion when Penny was in danger of being rumbled by Dorothy, they would both have needed to be implicitly seeing the conversation as a pretence, an exchange with inverted commas indicating it is 'as if', play, not for real. The difference is that verbal ping-pong is very much for real. Going back to Dorothy's discomfort with Penny's comment about the luggage, she needed to feel that Penny's fascination and approval were not simulated, and that she was making sense. Having to think fast in order to get the game back on track, Penny said, 'Silly me! You're right!' and discovered that this was all that was needed for her mother to feel in control again. Dorothy quickly resumed the illusion, saying confidently, 'That's why we always fly Swiss Air.'

Dorothy needed to know that she was holding Penny's attention in an authentic way and was quick to know when she was not. The person with dementia is storing feelings all the time, and those feelings will pick up anything from the carer that is contrived or artificial. Penny secured the save with the 'silly me' solution and as ever, the amber turned straight back to green. Nor was it inauthentic. What Penny felt when saying this was, 'Silly me, I've gone to sleep on the job, and the only thing that matters here is that in no way does my mother think she is being boring or a nuisance. Her well-being depends on my ability to reassure her that she is doing fine.' So however much pretence is required for ping-pong, the client will always pick up your authentic desire to help them, the love that lies behind the game, and it is this which authenticates it and gives you consent to play.

'My mother has only two stories in her repertoire, which she loves telling. I am worried that I ought to be getting her to talk about something different. How can I stop her repeating so much?'

Now that you have learned to play ping-pong you will know that safe, old pages are the bedrock of the SPECAL method. Contrary to common sense, in SPECALSENSE a great deal of repetition is not at all a bad thing.

For example, a carer told Penny about the worrying way in which her mother repeated the same story when they were together in the car. The story centred on a time when the client had managed to inflict a wound on her fencing instructor, while still a schoolgirl. She regaled her daughter with this saga 30 times in one journey. In the hope of inspiring some plot development, at first her daughter tried asking for details about the event: 'Had there been any blood?', 'Was this in the school gym?', 'Did the instructor cease teaching her?'

When this failed, she tried distractions: 'Look at those people at that bus stop', 'The weather seems to be getting worse', 'I wonder what we should have for supper.' Alas, nothing stemmed the flow or led to new details, it was always the same information delivered in the same way, seemingly for the first time.

SPECALSENSE rejects asking questions as a strategy because the client would have to stop and think. She would be unable to track back to where she had been before the interruption and would therefore tend to start all over again at the beginning. Rather than interrupt, why not just let her mother enjoy the benign activity of story telling? After all, if this was a child who was regaling you with the same stories you would cut them a lot of slack.

The difference between a carer's frustration about client repetitiveness and their tolerance in the face of children's repetitiveness is striking. Many parents will repeatedly reread stories in response to cries of 'again, again' from their little angel, without despair or irritation, sometimes enjoying the child's enthusiasm. Yet when it comes to a client who is repeating a story or question, if experienced from the normal position of common sense that most of us inhabit for most of the time, it is hard not to feel negative. That children adore repetition is illustrated by the decision on the part of the makers of Teletubbies to instantly replay the little stories from real life that they include as part of the programme. Incredibly to an adult, a small child will sit enchanted, while a story they have just seen about visiting a farm or building a boat is repeated. The repetitiveness of clients often seems equally incomprehensible but we find it considerably less endearing. Along with ping-pong, the next chapter offers a technique which will transform your attitude to client repetition.

But before proceeding to it, you need to go and practice your ping-pong. Don't forget to only do it in blocks of 10 minutes, at first, gradually building it up. It's hard work to start with but gets easier and easier as you practice. Only when you can establish a decent game should you read on. The steps required to play are summarised as follows:

TO PLAY VERBAL PING-PONG WITH A CLIENT

1. Choose a topic from earlier pages in their album. Select from areas of previous strength, happiness or expertise, at work or home.

2. Start limbering up with general prattle:

- The weather
- Your clothes
- Chores
- Cooking
- Shopping
- Anything that comes to mind

3. Lob over the first ball. If it does not come back, keep lobbing it, observing closely to see how different ways of positioning it get greater or lesser degrees of interest. Be very persistent, constantly seeking new ways of doing it. Some sentence stems you might like to try are:

- Perhaps . . .
- I suppose . . .

- I wonder whether/why/ how/when, etc . . .
- Some people say . . .
- I've heard that . . .
- I can't imagine why/how/when/where/why, etc . . .

4. As soon as a ball comes back over the net, give it a gentle return, whatever the subject, however it has been presented, exuding over-the-top enthusiasm:

- How fascinating/interesting/revelatory/weird/surprising!
- No! You're pulling my leg! Never!
- I'd never have guessed/known/worked that out/sussed that out!
- Amazing/stunning/brilliant/fabulous/excellent!
- Everything falls into place now/makes sense/seems clearer!

5. Note the precise words that the client has used and play them back verbatim after a brief pause.

6. Mirror their delivery:

- Speed
- Timing
- Timbre
- Body position
- Hand gestures
- Nonsense rhyme particular words

7. Match their body language, staying in tune on the emotional level as much as possible.

8. Once the rally is up and running, use the minimum to keep it going:

- Nods
- Single words
- Mmm, hmm, etc.
- Raised eyebrows
- Smile

When the rally is under way, be the first to show signs of needing refreshment and gently cue in a cup of tea, or some other therapeutic distraction, as you return from your game of the past to the routine activities of the present day. Stop while the client is on green, before they begin to fatigue of the game and allow them to support you – the less competent, more unfit player!

CHAPTER FIVE

Learn from the Expert

Until they understand the SPECAL approach, most carers groan with boredom and perplexity at the tendency of clients to endlessly repeat the same old questions. What you need to understand is that these questions are also the bane of the client's life. They reflect a nagging anxiety that signals amber and calls for a particular SPECAL technique as the best response. It provides you with the best answer to the question and then you can, courtesy of dementia, repeat that answer to the same question again and again. You will learn to love the repetition because you have found an answer that works.

If a client continues to ask the same anxious question again and again, it is obvious the best answer has yet to be found – no point you repeating the same common sense one if it's not reassuring. Perhaps you've given up answering anyway, as the client is failing to store what you say.

For example, a client had an utterly predictable series of questions that would arise as soon as it was time to leave the house: where is my hat/coat/purse/umbrella? As the illness got worse, it took her daughter longer and longer to get them both out the door. Then, when finally halfway down the stairs, the mother would suddenly decide it was time to change her lipstick colour. Her daughter found herself having to start planning for a departure one and a half hours beforehand. She would then give her mother a countdown: 30 minutes, 15 minutes, 1 minute, but it made no difference. 'Why didn't you tell me we are going out?' would come the question, however much warning had been provided.

This chapter offers a technique for enabling the carer to become as pleased by client repetition as parents are by their children's. Implausible though it may seem, repetition is a major source of well-being for clients and once you get it working for you, it soon becomes a lifeline. It is just a matter of finding out exactly what you need to repeat.

So why do clients repeat questions so much? It is invariably because they need information. Sometimes the quest takes the form of actually wandering about, physically setting off in search of an answer. But it is always at heart a matter of mental searching. Constantly asking the same question may be because they have a specific fear – as in, 'Where is my husband? I feel defenceless without him' – or it may reflect a lack of confidence because they realise they are liable to forget things – as in, 'Where's my purse? I don't want to go out without any money.' Either way, the client is asking for information that they currently need and cannot at that moment find.

To understand why repetition is a key to well-being you need to know the four basic conditions regarded as essential for that desirable state, regardless of whether you have got dementia.[8]

---

[8] Kitwood, T., 1997, *Dementia Reconsidered: The Person Comes First*, Buckingham: OUP.

1. Personal worth, the feeling that one is valued by oneself and others. We all need to feel valuable.

2. A sense of control, authority and agency. Agency is an important word that means feeling in control of one's personal life, being able to make decisions and ensure they are implemented.

3. Social ease. We have to be able to initiate contact and get a response from others, and to feel at ease about sharing social space.

4. Following from the presence of the first three basic conditions, we need to have trust and confidence that all will be well in the end, whatever happens, a kind of failsafe optimism to fall back on.

Formulated like that, only a moment's thought makes you realise why dementia so threatens client well-being. Clients are constantly reminded of their lack of value, as they find themselves cursing their inability to recall basic facts of their life and as others manifestly overrule them where once they would have been the first port of call for advice. Their agency and authority is removed summarily from them – the government takes away their driving licence, their carer tells them not to bother helping with the washing up because it will take five times longer if they participate and to leave the ironing for fear they will burn the house down. Their ease regarding initiating conversation with and responding to others collapses when they find themselves adrift halfway through a sentence whose beginning they cannot recall. They find themselves subtly cold-shouldered as people avoid even trying to start conversations. Most distressing of all, these repeated experiences lead them inexorably towards the opposite of a confidence that all will be for the best – this failsafe conviction is replaced by a black pessimism as to what the future holds.

But if clients are losing these pillars of well-being like skittles in a bowling alley, things are often only marginally better for the carer. Not a lot of feelings of self-worth come from being yacked at all day by an unreceptive, unsupportive client, and all too often, no one else seems to notice that you are busting a gut to try and keep them from falling apart. Your sense of agency is hardly enhanced by finding that your best efforts seem to do nothing to help the client: you feel out of control. Your need for convivial company is not provided by the client yet your social circle is liable to contract as visitors become less frequent, often too frightened by the changes in the client (dementia always poses the chilling question – 'and what if that were me?'). You are so busy keeping the client going that little time or energy is left for anyone else. When you repeat this scenario for months and months, turning into years, it is no wonder that you feel desperate when asked to picture the future.

And yet it really does not need to be like this. While all clients present a huge challenge to their carers' sanity, there is a simple method for dealing with the grinding repetition and the daily behavioural problems, one which turns them on their head, changing the situation from one of personal hell to salvation. Penny Garner calls this method SPOT.[9] It teaches you how to identify the repetitive and troublesome patterns, addresses any underlying anxieties and converts them into well-being for you both. It is very simple.

[9] Strictly speaking, this is an acronym: SPECAL Observational Tracking. It was developed by Penny Garner and influenced by Professor Tom Kitwood of Bradford University, who devised a monitoring tool called Dementia Care Mapping.

HOW TO SPOT

Draw a line down the middle of a page in your notebook. On the left-hand side, write a list of the questions that your client is liable to ask, each on a different line, sticking as closely as possible to the actual words they use. For one day, listen out for the number of times they ask these questions and put a cross against the relevant question in the right-hand column.

It is important not to actually make the notation in the company of the client. You are embarking on an activity related to the client's dementia and we must avoid any unnecessary focus on the illness when in their company. They have quite enough awareness of the problem from within themselves, without any additional reminder from their companions. So you are going to have to simply keep a mental note and then, when opportunity knocks, go and make an entry in your book. Alternatively, if you have an explanation of your activity which is wholly acceptable to the client, you might be able to jot something down on a piece of paper at the time. For example, if they are used to you doing a crossword you can scribble alongside: the activity of jotting down words will be perfectly in keeping with what you are doing. You will be able to capture the client's precise words and transfer them to your book later on.

By the end of the day you will have a picture of which question is the most repeated. For example, they may have asked most frequently, 'What's Andrew doing?' (let's suppose Ted is your husband and Andrew is your grown-up son), then 'Where is my book?', then 'Where are my glasses?' and then 'Shall I make some soup?'

Now take another page of your book and copy out the first of the most frequently asked questions at the top (in the example from above it was 'What's Andrew doing?'). Draw a line down the middle of the page and on the left-hand side make a list of possible answers. In composing these, you are searching for the one that will be most acceptable to the client. Without getting too fussy, try and dream up as many as you can. For example, if it were the Andrew scenario, you might put 'Andrew's playing tennis', 'Andrew's popped out for a moment', 'Andrew's gone to the shops', 'Andrew's at the dentist' and so on. Always include the name of the person the enquiry refers to, and keep the answer very short and simple. You may start by writing 'Andrew's gone to the shops to get some more beer because we've run out.' That sentence contains three possible answers: 'the shops', 'the beer' and 'because we've run out'. Each should appear separately on your list. You need to make the information in each answer concise and simple.

Given that the client (your husband) is referring to your son, you must consider the possibility that they are not necessarily referring to the Andrew of the present day. So in your list you should include plenty of possibilities from the past as well: 'doing something at school', 'playing football', 'he's at the cinema', 'out with his girlfriend'; actual scenarios from the past. In composing this list of possibilities, the more you can be guided by comments the client may have made about Andrew in recent times, the better. If there are clues that they are referring to the Andrew who is at university rather than at school, then go down that road, if it's the Andrew of early childhood, then that can be pursued. Just make an informed guess at the possibilities of what is going to be the most interesting and pleasurable one for the client.

Having SPOTted this list of answers, number them in order of which you believe is most likely to seem acceptable to the client. Now you can test your predictions. Over the next day, or days, whenever the client asks, 'What's Andrew doing?' try out an answer from your list, starting with the one you expect to be most acceptable and not giving up until you have tried them all. Observe closely how the client responds to each and give a score between 1 and 10, in terms of how much well-being seems to have resulted from that answer. You may think you have hit the nail on the head with the first answer and give it a 10, but do not stop at that because you might be surprised by getting even more benign reactions to subsequent ones. Once you have found the answer which rates the best, that is the one you should use. It is likely to work over and over again, a relief to both of you.

For example, in the case of the lady who could not leave the house without asking questions, if the best answer to the initial question, 'Where's my hat?' could be found, further similar questions about coat, purse and umbrella would be unlikely to arise. It turned out that the mother was principally worried about her appearance. Addressing this anxiety by using the particular phrase, 'This is a hat-free day. What a relief. We've got everything we need!' won. It took the daughter quite a lot of work in her notebook to find the best answer but once she found it and started using it all the time, their departure was never delayed.

Essential for SPOTting is that you become highly skilled at discerning the client's reaction. Obviously, if they respond to your answer with a furious shout of 'Andrew's a lazy boy, he's always been late', then it's probably a 1, and if it's greeted with a peaceful, happy smile and, 'Ah, that's good news. Nice to know he's all right', then it's likely to score a 10. But most of the reactions may not be so clear-cut. A brief exercise on yourself quickly exposes the subtleties of the problem of working out what they are thinking and feeling.

Try listing in your notebook the particular ways in which you indicate to someone that you are feeling positive or negative about what is going on around you – not just the ones everyone uses, like laughing or grimacing, but also record the idiosyncrasies. When I was asked I wrote down the following signs of negativity: knotted eyebrows, stroking upper lip, looking at floor, seeing without seeing (blank stares), furious denunciation of the world ('it's outrageous', 'it's truly disgraceful' and so forth). Signs that I am in a positive state include imitating others' voices, and nodding and putting my head to one side as I listen with a captivated expression. But even these are blunt, crude tools with which to unpick the complexities of my mood. I may be smiling, but sometimes that's to stop me snarling. I may be denouncing the latest atrocious announcement by our government, but doing so might be giving me a lot of pleasure. Only people who know me very well can really tell my positives and negatives, the behaviour alone is not enough. My wife or sisters or close friends are sufficiently knowledgeable about what rings my bell for good or ill, to be able to put my nodding or knotting eyebrows into context. Nonetheless, once you get to know me, there are some pretty reliable signs, whether it's just that I want to go and slump in front of the telly (surefire sign of exhaustion or mild depression) or that I want a drink (actually quite rare, nearly always a sign of a good mood – and that's before the drink).

Having listed your own indicators, now try doing the same for your client. The more you think about it, the more you realise that there are some basic and consistent patterns. For the negatives, carers list things like dragging of feet when walking, eyes going blank, acting as if stunned after a fall or a bang on the head, constantly asking the same question, wandering aimlessly and becoming very anxious that something urgently needs dealing with. Regarding positives, they list full eye-contact being made, beaming smiles and laughing, relaxed posture, humming a tune and active observation around the room or through a window.

In general, people with dementia, depending on how advanced

the illness is and the kind of care they have had, are liable to have a lot of negative signs. By far the most worrying is a grey, spectral complexion and demeanour, in which there is no eye-contact, the face blankly expressionless, almost catatonic. Yet there are sometimes spectacular shifts out of this state within seconds, as abrupt and transformative as the sun coming out from behind a cloud on a summer's day. When awoken from virtual somnambulance by a connection with photographs from early in their album, perhaps as far back as their childhood, they are unrecognisably different: talkative, flowing, shining, their face animated and as full of life as they ever were. Yet it can be a matter of seconds before the sun goes in again. As one carer put it, his wife could be in full flow and then suddenly she would worry where her purse had gone. This single moment of doubt could throw her into a state of extreme perplexity for the rest of the day, for she can shift from the purse location to a series of further questions to which no answers are stored: Why do I need my purse? Why do I not know why I need it? Rapidly, panic grows, overriding everything else. It has got to be sorted out, now, but she feels she has lost that basic sense of control. Perhaps her purse is a crucial indicator to her of who she is, even her very name. It is completely terrifying to realise that you do not know who you are and that purse must be found at all costs, immediately.

There is a lot at stake when it comes to being able to read the client's state. The more that you are able to develop a clear idea of the clues, the more you will be able to anticipate problems or, if they arise, the better able to provide remedies. What is more, once highly developed, your knowledge becomes transferable to other carers. Eventually, when properly briefed and after they have also digested this book, other carers can be enabled to take a significant part of the care burden off your shoulders.

FROM SPOTTING TO VERBAL PING-PONG

If we go back to Ted's question 'What's Andrew doing?', the best answer eventually selected by his wife was 'Andrew's out playing football.' This produced a sigh of pleasure from Ted because he had always been very proud of his son's success in this sport. Ted's carer had to stay alert because just occasionally he would look puzzled by the reply and provide a follow-on question. The carer had to be ready to supply additional information if required. Sometimes Ted would say, 'Football again? Surely he gets enough practice – does he have to keep playing?' and the carer then needed to explore what the best follow-on answer might be. This turned out to be 'Andrew often helps out with the juniors' as Ted approved of his teaching others as well as playing himself. What was most important was the way in which his wife managed to combine verbal ping-pong with the carefully tested answer to sustain a recurrent satisfactory state for the client, no matter how many follow-on questions were asked.

Luckily for his wife, football was one of Ted's conversational favourite topics for verbal ping-pong (as it would be for me!). They had developed a very satisfactory rally in which the ping-pong ball was Ted's finest hour playing as a goalkeeper in his school team. Once the subject was underway, Ted only needed an occasional gesture of reaching out as if to catch a football or muttering the word 'penalty' to keep on going quite happily. It is not hard to see that when his wife identified that being 'out playing football' was the best answer to the question of Andrew's whereabouts she quickly realised she was onto another winner for verbal ping-pong. It took only a bit more SPOTting to work out which of Andrew's footballing successes lit Ted up. Having tried out several occasions when Ted had witnessed Andrew score goals, his wife identified a particular header, and ever afterwards, they had a safe, highly satisfying sequence:

> TED: Where's Andrew gone?
> HIS WIFE: He's out playing football.
> *Pause, as client looks pleased.*
> HIS WIFE: Ah, he really can head a football, can Andrew.
> TED: Headers . . . that reminds me of the day . . .
> *and he embarks on his own reminiscences of football.*

On reading this, some carers may imagine that I have taken leave of my senses. The inference would appear to be that it is desirable to encourage clients to repeat the same stories. Since this is exactly the conversational dead end from which most carers are trying to escape, it is easy to see why you might think I am mad. But before you ring for the men in white coats, backtrack a moment.

The photograph album analogy explains how the core problem faced by someone with dementia is lack of information on present pages. All their difficulties stem from this disability. Without it they would be exactly the same as they would otherwise have been. The SPECAL method is designed to minimise the danger of reds arising from the client's blanks. This is achieved by creating 24-hour wraparound care that protects them from ever needing to rely on new information. By turning to the early pages with old memories, where there are no blanks and linking these to the activities of daily life today, they are able to live in a wholly safe place.

If you follow the logic, then you can see that repetition of happy stories is not only safe, it is happy too. While that is not all there is to the SPECAL method, this is its core: helping the client throughout their waking hours to access reliably happy memories and to use these as a substitute for more recent information that is either missing or gravely impaired. Verbal ping-pong is the starting point for achieving this, by identifying favourite topics from the past to play with. SPOTting is a way of pinpointing the day-to-day anxieties and problems which recur for the client and having done so, of providing acceptable explanations and answers. Put the two together and the acceptable answers derived from SPOTting can be added to the cache of balls for playing verbal ping-pong.

In the case of 'Where's Andrew gone?', putting the two together was unusually easy because one of the client's favourite topics (football) overlapped with the acceptable answer to his repeated question (gone to play football). In other cases, the answer and the topic may ostensibly be unconnected. For instance, suppose the three favourite topics are the famous Christmas episode of *EastEnders* in 1986 when Den told Angie he wanted a divorce; knitting; and walking in the park. Suppose the question was 'Where's my purse?' and the acceptable answer 'Don't worry, if we go out I'll make sure I've got some money on me.' On the face of it, the favourite topics and the answers are quite different. In fact, this is almost never the case: with very little imagination you can always find a link. Perhaps you can see a way to link up one of these topics to this answer.

Suppose you have just given that answer ('I've got some money') to the repeated question as to the whereabouts of the purse. If it's something that you used to do, or still do, you might say 'I've got money if we go out to the pub.' You might add 'funny how *EastEnders* always seems to go on in that pub. The Queen Vic.' Sure enough, you have made it back to the favourite topic.

Or regarding knitting, after giving the acceptable answer you might add, 'We might want to go out later to buy some wool for your knitting', if the client still does knitting or talks about doing it. Or regarding going to the park, after the acceptable answer you might add, 'I'll take some money if we go out to the park later.'

This might sound awfully tricksy but it is not nearly as elaborate as that. Just give it a try. Write down your client's three favourite topics. Now write down the acceptable answer to their commonest repeated question. Now let your imagination do the rest . . . see what I mean?

SPECALSENSE is actually quite fun once you get into the habit. Hard though it may be to believe, instead of finding yourself trapped with a stuck gramophone record, verbal ping-pong and SPOTting can make being with the client an endless source of fascination and enjoyment. Not only will you learn to love repetition, you will also see that it vastly improves client well-being and therefore, yours as well. Consider this final example.

One of Mary's most frequently asked questions of Paul was 'What did you say?' Paul came to see, quite quickly, when he employed SPECALSENSE, that offering the answer, 'I didn't say anything' was about as stultifying to Mary as it could possibly be. It was a prime example of how *not* to play verbal ping-pong, as good as hitting the ball way out of her reach and completely out of play. When he began trying out various other answers, over several months, he came up with one or two that scored reasonably well, and Mary seemed passably content with his offering. But the questions continued to come and Paul still felt he hadn't found the best answer yet. Then he found a real winner, the statement they both needed.

They were sitting together in a comfortable silence when Mary said, 'What did you say?' Paul, in a moment of inspiration (mainly triggered by having run out of any ideas), looked tenderly at her and said, 'I was thinking how much I love you.' This was perhaps the first time that Paul understood how simple SPECAL can become, provided it is authentic. From that day onwards, Mary's repeated question ceased to be a problem. They had both learned to love it.

TROUBLESHOOTING

'Won't it be intolerably dull for me to have to listen to the same story again and again?'

As a carer you may find it tough already but the prospect of having a client who is stuck on a permanent loop of telling the same story all day long could seem even worse. Panic not. A major objective of developing favourite topics for ping-pong and of SPOTting acceptable answers is to be able to provide transferable skills, so that soon you can safely leave the client with other people. This is explained further in subsequent chapters. As outlined above, no one can sustain well-being as a carer if they do nothing else. Carers with ill-being are not only going to be miserable, they are not going to be providing very good care. It is a crucial component of the 24-hour wraparound method that it can be provided by a succession of changing carers, once you have all the necessary components in place, of which favourite topics and acceptable answers are the first two. Eventually, when the illness progresses to the later stages, Penny strongly advocates the transfer of the client to a nursing home, on the basis that this will be in the best interests of the client. At a certain point, and sooner than many people realise, the client thrives on spending time with other people with dementia. The best companion for a person with dementia is another one, provided that the staff are interested in wraparound care and properly briefed by the carer. So be reassured, you are not being condemned to the same fate as the central character in Evelyn Waugh's novel A *Handful of*

Dust who was trapped in the Brazilian jungle with a madman who forces him to reread Charles Dickens novels for the rest of his life.

You may already have noted that playing ping-pong and SPOTting are fascinating and rewarding. Far from being passive and bored when the client is repeating their story, you will be constantly looking for ways to keep the game going, for new revelations by the client and for inventive ways to link to practical, everyday life – see next problem.

'If I encourage them to get locked into the past, how am I ever going to get them to do any of the everyday things, like go to bed or brush their hair?'
If all SPECAL was doing was teaching you how to encourage your client to reminisce about their past, that would not be enough. The answer is provided in later chapters but fear not, both favourite topics and acceptable answers can be used to enable usually very tricky vital daily activities to become effortless.

'Am I going to have to turn into a cracked record myself? Will the client notice that I'm turning into a new form of deranged parrot?'
To get alongside a client you must offer what they need. The repetition you are learning to learn to love is of what works for them. The client is storing all feelings and you are aiming to find the answer that generates the maximum relief and satisfaction. With each repetition you increase the chances that the question will gradually fade away because the anxiety behind it is being dealt with by the acceptable answer. When that happens, you move on to the next question and find the most acceptable answer for that. In due course you will iron out most, if not all, of the questions that cause the client anxiety.

'I have tried playing ping-pong with my wife, but she is far too busy asking about where her mother is. What am I doing wrong?'

Start SPOTting your wife's questions about her mother, and decide which the most frequent question is. Then use verbal ping-pong to introduce gentle chat about her mother, as you explore what the answer to the question should be. During the course of these conversations you will uncover new insights which will help you allay other anxieties. You will soon be playing fluent ping-pong without nearly so many interruptions.

'What do I do if the client keeps repeating a story that causes them great distress?'

There is a particular way of dealing with this situation. The device you need is the Red-to-Green Conversational Loop described in detail in the next chapter.

SPOTTING

1. Write down on the left-hand side of a page in your notebook the most common questions that the client asks.

2. Observe for a day, noting down the number of times each question is asked beside it on the right.

3. On a new sheet of paper, taking the most frequently asked question, write down all the answers you can think of that might be acceptable to the client, bearing in mind that they may refer to long-distant events in the past.

4. Put numbers by each of the answers, guessing which will be the most acceptable.

5. Taking the one you believe is most likely to be accepted first, give a score from 1 to 10 of how much the answer promoted well-being in the client. Then work through all the remaining answers in your list.

CONVERT THE ANSWER INTO A FAVOURITE TOPIC FOR PING-PONG

1. Write down the three favourite topics for verbal ping-pong that you chose in the last chapter.

2. Write down the answer that was most acceptable to the most repeated question.

3. Let your mind float freely in finding links between the answer and the topics.

Now you are well prepared for the next time the question is asked. You are equipped with the best possible answer and also the all-important link into a safe, meandering pathway of therapeutic conversation. The value of carer confidence in the face of the client's most frequently asked questions cannot be overstated. Your gentle air of conveying good news and happy cues will lead to a remarkable reduction of anxious repetition from the client and a better life for you both.

CHAPTER SIX

NEVER CONTRADICT

After 'don't ask questions' and 'learn from the expert', the SPECAL third commandment is 'never contradict' (the client). To be precise, Penny Garner advocates counting to three and then agreeing, or at least not disagreeing. During the pause, suspend any immediate, common sense disagreement that you may have with what they are saying and indicate, however tacitly, that they are right. It is crucial to be convinced and convincing, so although you disagree with them factually, remind yourself that there is a higher-order consideration behind your agreement: you are passionately committed to the client's well-being. If you merely confirm something verbally that you actually disagree with, your body language will be out of sync with the words. The feeling of disagreement will be picked up, so in the pause remind yourself of your concern for the client. Feelings are more important than facts and you must avoid discord on the feelings front, whatever the facts.

That raises an immediate problem for many carers: 'I'm sorry, I cannot bring myself to lie to my spouse/partner/parent. If they say something that I know to be untrue, I really can't go along with it because it totally betrays the bond of trust and honesty which we have built up over the years. How can I authentically agree to something I disagree with?' Penny's robust retort is that the carer must grow up and take responsibility. If they really want to protect their client from reds and provide wraparound care, then they must do everything necessary to avoid new factual information, and that means not imposing present-day reality unnecessarily. If the client believes themselves to be in an airport lounge in 1973 awaiting a flight to Athens, when we believe them to be in a nursing home in 2008, to insist on the 2008 version would be immature and selfish as well as destructive, says Penny. Although she does not use the analogy, I would further ask whether you would deliberately impose adult reality on a small child's fantasy. If it is time for bed during a six-year-old's game involving Father Christmas, you might adapt the fantasy to get the child upstairs quickly and happily, as the big man likes children to be asleep when he visits. Few parents would resort to insisting that he doesn't exist. So if you are prepared to allow your children their illusions, why are you so insistent that your client's must be exposed?

Penny's key point about avoiding disagreement with clients is that you can use the disability to mutual advantage. Even if the client says they are going to do something that is potentially disastrous, like take the car for a ride or leave the nursing home right now, both your interests and theirs will be served by avoiding any disagreement about the *facts* at that moment. If you can foster well-being *feelings*, like autonomy, it will be easier by far to negotiate with them in a moment's time. That means you can and must avoid direct confrontational disagreement with them over anything they say, at the point when they say it. Provided you do not disturb their sense that they are doing okay at that moment, then, in the next moments after the statement (at which point they are already losing the facts of what has just been said) you can move on.

Does that make you uneasy? If so, when honestly considered, you will see this is a problem in you, not your client.

Your first objection is liable to be that it will betray the bond of trust; you feel you will be lying to them. Behind this may be a reluctance to face the reality of the disability that your client has developed, as it's just too painful to acknowledge that this person will never be the same as they once were and 'giving in' or 'pandering' to what you see as their illusions, treating them like a child, is too painful. By now, having read thus far, hopefully you are realising that a lot of the adult person you once knew in the client is in fact still there and waiting to communicate with you if you can find the right methods.

But equally distressing, you have to overcome your natural reluctance to comply with a version of reality that you may regard as more or less bonkers. If you dig deep enough, you will soon see that, first and foremost, your urge to assert that your reality is the true one is in order to keep yourself from feeling you are going bonkers too, to protect yourself, not the client. The reason you are currently providing to yourself or others may be that you need to help the client to 'stay in touch with reality', or some such. The truth is that you are scared to allow their version because it threatens your sanity. And that is why Penny responds with the almost derogatory injunction to grow up. She means that you are losing track of the real situation here, which is that you are the one who is still storing new information, the one without the disability, and you must take responsibility for the client, as they would be sure to ask you to, were it possible to put the scenario to them. I would add that just as a parent must take responsibility for their child – because parents know a lot of stuff children do not – so with carers and clients. Very often, anyway, it's a case of not disagreeing, a passive mode which requires no actual steering.

In return for agreeing (or just not disagreeing) you will instantly be heading towards greener psychological pastures. Bearing in mind Penny's list of the prerequisites for well-being (agency, social ease and so on), agreement increases feelings of being valued, especially if it is done using praise and admiration, however much you may be feeling their opposites, at least to begin with. Saying 'What a super idea, you have such good ideas about what we should do' when your client suggests having supper only a minute after you have cleared it away; saying 'Brilliant, how fascinating' when your client repeats an opinion with which you have always strongly disagreed; or saying 'Wow, that's amazing' if the client tells you that they are about to close a deal worth a lot of money, referring to something that happened 20 years ago; doing these things all make the client feel good about themselves. Equally, such reactions may increase their sense of agency and authority. They are the boss, they know what's what, they are not the hopeless wreck with a failing memory that they may fear. Agreeing also opens up the field for further chat, creating the feeling of being part of a social world in which they communicate and others communicate back, contingently. Taken together, these create a secure, contented state of mind that feeds into the conviction that everything will be all right. Never forget that feelings and non-verbal communication are much more important to the client than normal, and they become ever more so as the illness progresses. Never mind the facts, feel the feelings – that must be your motto.

You may be wondering how far this has to be taken. Is it seriously being contended that the carer should agree with absolutely everything the client says? Incredible though it may seem, the answer is yes but only in the sense that you must not actively *disagree*. That does not mean you will stay in the same place for ever: as noted, you can afford to agree because the dementia can be relied upon to work for you. For instance, a carer's mother had started hallucinating insects, really seeing them moving about, even making friends with them as pets. The delusions were not in themselves symptoms of dementia but SPECALCARE required that they be incorporated into the package. One evening, the client took the carer out to the garden to look at the insects: 'See them? They gather in the evening as it gets dark, they prefer it on the steps near the house because it's warmer.' The carer did not agree but she did not disagree either. She commented 'how interesting' and then picked up a leaf that was lying at the point where her mother believed there was an insect. Knowing the client very well, the carer was aware that she had an encyclo-paedic knowledge of different trees and said, 'Ah look, here's an oak leaf, and this one's a hawthorn, I think.' The client looked at it and said, 'Yes, that's right, a hawthorn' without any problem at all because her daughter had successfully opened the old pages where knowledge of leaves were stored. This opening of useful, old green pages is only possible when the client is feeling confident and secure, not battered by disagreement.

Alas, all too often problems are created by people not aware of the SPECAL approach. A carer had a client wife who was convinced that their son's marriage was deeply troubled when, as far as the carer knew, it was nothing of the sort. When advised that he should agree with everything the client says, he could just about imagine doing so when they were on their own, but surely it was not right to confirm a blatant untruth in front of other people, some of whom might gossip? Penny responded that the key was preparation. So long as everyone who came into contact with the client was carefully briefed in advance it would be fine. He should explain that the client has a disability that sometimes leads to potentially problematic events, like repetition of stories or saying things which seem to other people either odd or untrue. Details need to be supplied, 'She is convinced our son's marriage is troubled. Just don't contradict her' or 'If she says there are large insects in front of her, don't worry about it, just don't disagree.' There is an obvious risk of sounding partronising or of making the visitors think it is embarrassing or pathetic that the client needs this kind of consideration. But that should not deter you because if you manage to sound positive and enthusiastic, the chances are they will enter into the spirit of what is going on. In the SPECAL view, if the client experiences a problem, it is ultimately being created by the way the people around them are responding, it's not actually in the client at all.

This was neatly illustrated by a problem a carer had when making visits to the theatre with his client wife. She would have no compunction in declaring in a loud voice that 'The costumes are just dreadful!' The carer could not see how to avoid saying 'Shhhh', creating a fuss and enraging his wife. Penny suggested arriving early so that he could chat to the people in nearby seats, explaining the situation briefly before the performance started. The carer tried this out, discreetly informing the other audience members that the client had a disability. He hoped they would not be too disturbed if she made the occasional rather loud remark. Of course, an acceptable explanation for the client was needed as to why the carer was chatting to surrounding people rather than to her. In this instance it was simple because the carer's profession was that of an Oxford city guide and the client used to accompany him on trips. When the client looked at him quizzically in the theatre, he simply pointed to the surrounding audience and said 'They need guiding – I'm just helping out.' The audience was sympathetic, he felt relaxed and this transmitted to the client. Interestingly, her wish to criticise during performances has virtually disappeared.

In other cases, it should always be possible to dream up something similar that will make sense to the client in terms of past history. In doing so, you are no more lying than when you tell your six-year-old child that Father Christmas will be delivering presents on a sleigh. It is a benign illusion, not a self-serving deceit: SPECALSENSE.

A good deal of having to agree with clients can be avoided just by not pursuing problematic lines of conversation. One client was liable to get extremely anxious about her daughter's visits. The daughter would call up and say 'I am coming to visit on Monday, Mum.' Her mother would say 'I must go and get my diary,' prompting a frantic, 'No, Mother, don't do that.' The daughter knew from past experience that her mother would consult her diary, get in a tizzy at a later hour and ring the daughter back, often several times a night, worrying that there was something she had forgotten. It would invariably turn out to be the visit. Sometimes these calls came at 2 a.m. and the daughter lived 40 miles away.

Penny's initial point to the daughter was that warning the mother of the precise facts of her forthcoming visit was in itself a mistake – it entailed new information which, whether written down or not, might not store in its entirety, if at all. But the feeling that something was about to happen would be stored, without the facts, and this might entail anxieties about duties to be fulfilled to make her guest happy. There was actually no point in advance warning other than immediately prior to arrival. A call on the mobile from the top of the street as the daughter arrived would work far better. That way, the pictures and the soundtrack would match.

The carer had a problem with this at first. Surely her mother would like to know she was coming, could make plans, could prepare? But as Penny pointed out, prepare for what? The facts of what she was meant to be preparing for would be lost, while the vague anxiety that she should be doing something would remain, which was triggering the 2 a.m. calls. The carer soon realised that her need to tell her mother about her forthcoming visit was the problem. Feeling guilty that she was unable to go more often, she wanted to give her mother the advance information to make herself feel better.

As the carer reflected further she uncovered a trove of reasons why her mother was generally anxious. Her mother had been a nurse in the war and she often referred to a matron who had terrorised her at that time. This seemed to connect to still earlier times when her mother had been sent away to a boarding school and been heavily punished if her uniform was not right or if her spelling or writing were not just so. This kind of background knowledge is incredibly important for being able to develop a fuller picture of what is going on in a client's mind and being able to provide acceptable explanations. It is also crucial for dealing with catastrophic reds. While I am reluctant to press further reading upon you, and especially so because it runs the risk of seeming like self-advertisement, you may possibly find it helpful to read my book *They F*** You Up*: it examines how family relationships affect us throughout life.

At least in the short-term, it's not hard to see how agreeing could increase harmony in relationships and client well-being. But you may still be troubled by those occasional situations where agreement would seem to run the risk of something disastrous happening right away. One carer's husband kept on insisting that they go for a drive and that, despite the fact that his licence had been taken away, he be the one to drive. His wife became deeply distressed by his rage when she refused to supply the car keys. He would scream and shout at her, frighteningly; yet if she agreed to the plan, surely he would kill them both? Penny confirmed that he should not be at the wheel. However, there were different ways of achieving that outcome, without upsetting him in the process. The carer wanted to know how, if he continued out of the door, keys in hand, could he possibly be stopped? She pointed out that her husband was quite a dictatorial man.

At the same group session, another carer reported that they had a client who needed physiotherapy but who refused to go because the therapist was 'Shit and they don't do it right and they're all bonkers at the clinic anyway.' If everyone just agreed with all this, how could anyone get the client to have the treatment? Penny's answer to these problems and to similar ones, is called the Red-to-Green Conversational Loop.

GETTING FROM RED TO GREEN

People with dementia can move very rapidly from green to red, only pausing briefly on amber. The upside of this febrility is that the reverse is also true – they can move with equal rapidity from red to green.

The first step away from red is for the carer to validate the client's experience by using every means at their disposal to make the client feel the carer is sharing the same emotions. Get alongside them, join their club and become a fully paid-up member – there are only two members, you and the client, and together you can take on the rest of the world. To validate, you have to draw on your own album and find a match as best you can to the feelings the client is demonstrating. If they are in a state of panic, so, in a sense, are you (you desperately need to help and don't know how). You shiver together as you share a frightening moment. You may not yet have the same understanding of why, but that is all about facts, and the facts will fall into place once the feelings have been addressed. Clearly the client is frightened about something, and you are frightened because they are frightened. You have the information from the client that the club to be joined is the 'we're two frightened people' club and that is your starting point.

One day, Jack, aged 72, was sitting enjoying a cup of coffee at the Day Unit in Burford. He was talking quite calmly to another person when suddenly, for no discernible reason, he dived under the table, sat on the floor and began shivering. The common sense response was to bend down and ask Jack if he was all right and to suggest he came out. This made Jack more agitated. Penny's validatory method was to drop something on the floor near the table and get on her knees so that she could shadow his behaviour while searching for what she had dropped. She was now down at his level, joining the 'we're both on the floor' club, which was at least a start. Having observed him shivering and clearly alarmed, Penny started shivering herself as she edged her way towards him under the table without directly engaging. She was literally and figuratively getting alongside him without picking up his gaze. She had no difficulty in being authentic about this, since she was feeling pretty apprehensive about how she was going to cope. Closely matching his body language (hands around knees, head turning to look around nervously), Penny casually caught his eye. He began to jabber away, fairly incomprehensibly, and Penny nodded. She looked across past the table legs as if wondering whether to move out. At once she caught a few words from Jack, 'It's not safe, we must stay here.' Penny nodded and said, 'You're right, I'm glad we've got each other, Jack', making it clear they were in it together, whatever 'it' was: at that moment it was the 'we're the shivering under the table' club and the 'we're the let's hope it'll soon be safe to come out' club.

Jack's confidence began to increase. She could see in his face that he was feeling less terrified and gradually was becoming more relaxed. She developed their relationship slightly more with 'Thank goodness you're here, Jack' and his sense of well-being visibly rose again as he felt of some use to her. She could begin the next stage of the Red-to-Green Conversational Loop – the stage known as 'flipping' from red to green, for which Penny needed more background information.

She chatted on, using her babbling technique, saying how awful it was and how she hoped things would get better soon. She looked at Jack from time to time, and then chanced a quick peer out from under the table. He immediately said, 'Be careful. We have to wait for the all-clear. It hasn't been sounded yet.' Penny nodded, her mind racing. All-clear – what could Jack mean? She thought back: who was Jack, before he got dementia? Oh yes, the facts she needed came to her, he had had a very difficult time in the war in North Africa. Now she knew what they were both up to, they were sheltering as they waited for the danger to pass overhead. So . . . while waiting for the next thing to happen, what more positive way could they find of spending the time? She searched for positive aspects of Jack's wartime experiences and a particularly favourite story of his came to her, one that she knew practically by heart. How he had somehow managed to squirrel away in his kitbag some silk stockings, which had bought him a few interesting favours on his way through Italy. She stretched out one stockinged leg and murmured that she hoped she hadn't laddered her stockings. She gave just a hint of showing a leg, a minute gesture which most people might have missed, but it was enough to trigger an immediate response in Jack, who said, with a wicked smile, 'Now, if you want to know a thing or two about stockings . . .' and he was off on his story, all shivering by now having completely disappeared.

The flip from red to green had been achieved but they were still under the table, caught up in the war. Penny knew instinctively that she needed something more to link the green to the reality of the present day before exiting from under the table. It was time to move into the final phase of the Red-to-Green Conversational Loop called the circuit-breaker, a dramatic mix of distraction and reality orientation delivered at speed. She needed to move Jack from North Africa to Burford and from war to peace, without giving him a huge shock, while he was still telling his story, still held in green.

Jack was at full narrative tilt. Penny peered out from under the table, clapped her hands very suddenly, tugging Jack's as she said with great urgency, 'Jack, quick! I've heard the all-clear and we mustn't miss our mug of tea!' Together they shot out, and as they did so Penny was already cueing in a reference to another Jack topic, the upholstering of armchairs. He knew a fair amount about that and its bounciness as a ping-pong ball was well proven.

The conversational looping from red to green can be thought of as a stopwatch showing 60 seconds. The clock starts ticking as Jack dives under the table. By the time the hand has reached quarter past, Penny is well into validation with Jack. She shares her thoughts about how worrying life is at the moment, taking care to ensure that nothing disturbs the sense that Jack is making of the situation. This is a far cry from the common sense idea of trying to persuade Jack to be sensible and come out from under the table and join everyone for lunch. Jack is reassured by the arrival of a fellow member of his current club, a club that, incidentally, Penny later learned had been created in the first place by the cook making a clanging noise with the saucepan lid in the kitchen next door. Penny encourages Jack to express the dangers and horrors of their situation with Penny nodding in agreement.

By the time the clock reaches the halfway mark, Penny has raised Jack's confidence level and pieced together enough information to flip the conversation from negative to positive recollections. Now she has moved Jack on to sufficient client green and can prepare to move, still using validation, into 'flipping'. It's a question of confidence and timing, like tossing a pancake, or a backwards swimming dive. It is a reversal, from 'Gosh how ghastly' to 'Golly, is there a redeeming feature?' You transfer the focus from negative to positive while remaining in the validated territory of old pages, which is where the red under review usually resides. Penny did it with Jack by cueing in the phrase 'silk stockings', reinforcing the connection by slightly raising her skirt. If common sense had been applied, by now Jack would have been left alone in the vain hope he would join everyone for lunch. Instead, he begins regaling Penny with a silk-stocking story. She coos with amazement at his feats, using vocabulary she knows he has used himself, ensuring that she remains tuned to his wavelength and offering no distractions. He has flipped into green, despite still being on 'war years' pages from his album.

You need enough biographical facts to place the client's negative feelings into some sort of context and you need to be silently, internally relating the facts of the situation as experienced by the client to this context. All the while, by being alongside your client, you are maintaining their sense of relief that they are not alone in their plight and offering the reassurance that comes from an injection of well-being.

By the time the clock has passed the three-quarters mark, it is time for the circuit-breaker. This reconnects the client to the contemporary context while sustaining their identity in an acceptable way. It is clear that Jack is securely held by his storytelling and Penny has the confidence to break the circuit of wartime experiences through a combination of sudden distraction followed immediately by orientation to a routine activity of daily life. Penny distracts through a sudden, loud clap of the hands, orientates by cueing in teatime (an activity of daily life, an important moment for anyone, and particularly a soldier) and validates by ushering Jack to an upholstered armchair which is a well-established prop supporting Jack's equally well-established topic of 'hospitality manager', a useful ball for verbal ping-pong. At the end of all this, Jack is completely restored to green.

The following week the same situation arose, but this time Penny was able to make the connection between the saucepan lids banging and Jack's sudden catapult under the table. By the week after, she had enough information to ensure that there was less saucepan clanging and at the sound of the merest tinkle, provided information to Jack that 'the cook is at it again!', pointing to the kitchen as she did so. By the fourth week, Jack's days in the air-raid shelter were over, never to return.

The common sense approach, expecting Jack to come out from under the table for a cup of tea without any validation of his air-raid plight, would not address Jack's red in any meaningful way. It would, at best, merely buy time before Jack returned to the silent wartime anguish. At worst, it would lead to resistance from Jack that might well turn into aggression and even violence. Eventually, the mental-health team might be called in, with referral to a specialist and medication for anxiety or psychosis prescribed. From the point of view of services, this would be expensive and undesirable. From Jack's point of view it would be disastrous: he would become groggy, his communication skills reduced and his long-term well-being severely compromised. In complete contrast, the Red-to-Green Conversational Loop provides a means of resolving the current red and opens the way to eliminating the risk of a similar episode arising again.

Of course, not all client reds are introduced on today's page by something as ordinary as the sound of a clanging saucepan lid. Many, indeed arguably most, reds have their origin in the potentially catastrophic experience of uncovering blanks in the album – of discovering that information which should have been stored simply does not exist. That is why the activity of consulting any page post-dementia carries such a huge risk for the client and why we, as carers, should avoid them at all costs. We should restrict ourselves to using repetitive old stuff that is known to be well book-marked, so to speak. We should also remember never to argue.

For example, a carer had left the client's supper for them in the fridge because she would not be back until later. On her return he said he had not eaten. When she went to the fridge there was nothing there and the carer (having already caused a potential problem by asking the question 'How was your supper?'), now said 'But I left you your supper and it's gone. You must have eaten it.' The client became extremely upset. How could the carer accuse him of lying? What did she think he was, an idiot who did not know if he'd eaten his supper? An argument developed and tempers were raised. He began to feel extremely anxious, vulnerable and hugely frustrated. He soon lost any connection with the facts that had triggered this outburst. Red blanks began to ribbon across his current page. The carer, in desperation, insisted that he come with her to the kitchen to see. Then he became even more disturbed because he saw the plate she had left for him when she went out. It was sitting on the sink with just a few bits of the supper remaining. She pointed out that this was his plate and he had eaten his supper after all. Having no photograph of any such event, he was frantically engaged on a fruitless search, so awash in red that he had no idea what she was talking about. Not only had he failed to store the fact that he had eaten his supper, but also the fact that supper was the matter under discussion.

The carer discussed this with Penny. Surely the only way forward was for her to give up her evening off, and stay in? She loved her husband dearly but was becoming terrified of his irrational outbursts. Penny suggested avoiding asking the client any questions when she returned from her evening off (a question had triggered the whole ghastly episode) and to adopt a combination of the 'don't disagree' and 'silly me!' tactics if she inadvertently triggered a similar situation in the future. Provided the client is not challenged and it is the carer who is silly rather than the client, most problems tend to fade away with extraordinary speed.

To validate, making the client feel they are being reasonable within their terms of reference, keep factual information to a minimum. This carer could say, 'Of course! Silly me! You're right!' The chances are that the client will be so relieved that they are not the silly one that all facts of the matter will become irrelevant as the feeling of green floods in. The carer can be ready with the follow-on, 'I seem to be all over the place these days. Just as well you're here to keep me right!' You, as the carer, now can use verbal ping-pong to get the conversation back on track, perhaps using that wonderful meal you shared many years ago, common to both your albums well before the onset of dementia. The phrase 'That reminds me . . .' is a wonderful carer tool to distract to green when used at the right moment.

Often the red has its origins in the fact that a person or object of significance is missing and the absence seems intolerable. For example, Sandra got in a terrible state about her handbag when staying in the hospital. It had been locked in the hospital safe with all her money while she was resident there. She found its constant absence from beside her chair incomprehensible and became really angry and almost paranoid about it, saying, 'Someone has stolen it. I shall have to report it to the police. Whatever place is this?' Rather than disagree and risk a further tirade, Penny set off together with her to search for the handbag, validating Sandra by muttering about how awful the place was, repeating her precise words. They became the 'fed up to the back teeth with this dreadful place' club and wandered out of the ward. Halfway down the corridor a nurse approached carrying a tea tray and looked at them enquiringly. Penny deliberately raised the tempo slightly, just above Sandra's level of outrage. 'We're looking for our handbags because we're absolutely fed up with it here. They must have been pinched.' Sandra immediately looked at Penny and said, in a slightly reproving way, 'It's not as bad as that you know.' In a flash, Sandra had switched from being the one who was persecuted to the great rescuer, the one in control, now swathed in green. The nurse was all set to explain about the handbag being in the hospital safe when Penny fixed her with a sharp look and explained again that they were both looking for their handbags. Sandra looked again at Penny and said 'You may be looking for a handbag dear, but I'm going to have a nice cup of tea.'

This illustrates how validation can be sufficient to move from red to green if combined with 'silly me'. When praise and encouragement are thrown in as well, it boosts the client's well-being and quite often their anxiety about missing people or objects evaporates. These anxieties reflect a mounting crisis in the client's life, on amber, but SPECALSENSE comes to the rescue.

To understand this better, you can perform a simple exercise:

think of the worst incident from your childhood when you felt utterly humiliated or abandoned or rejected. Penny's example is her first day at a new school when she was aged 11. A fearsome woman with a bun looked her up and down, with a piercing stare. Penny's mother had also attended the same school many moons before but the staff had clearly not changed that much and the teacher said, 'You look remarkably like Dorothy Stewart. I saw her daughter's name on the list. I hope you're not going to be anything like your mother. She was the untidiest child I have ever had to deal with.' The look of downright disdain and disapproval, before Penny had said a word, remains etched in her mind as one of the worst put-downs she has ever known. She felt she had been labelled as hopeless before her first term had begun.

If you consider your worst childhood scenario, what would have helped you to feel better at that moment? You can see that if someone had come alongside you, sympathising with the distress and sharing it as something they had suffered as well, it would have helped. If they had then covered you in praise and admiration for the skill with which you had helped them in some way, you could have recovered altogether from your distress.

Now you should do a further exercise.

EXERCISE: Anticipating the worst moment with the client (daily or occasional)

Identify the worst problem you encounter in caring for your client during a typical 24-hour period. It might be getting them to bed or keeping them from setting off in the car or that they get hyper-anxious for no apparent reason. It might be when they first wake up. Choose the worst you can think of and give it a title.

Examples from carers recently have included:

'The Hosepipe', when the client washes the car both inside and out; 'The TV Shutdown', when the carer wants to watch the news and the client becomes obsessed with trying to leave the house just as the news starts; and 'The Vest Reversal', when the client first puts on their vest, then takes it off, then starts again.

Now write down your title at the top of a page in your notebook and think what you could say that would validate the client in this situation. Try and think of a family phrase that might fit the bill. 'The Hosepipe' involved 'Nothing like a good drop of rain for bringing out the best'; 'The TV Shutdown': 'Well, it's goodnight from him . . .'; 'The Vest Reversal': 'Now we see it, now we don't.' All were well-known family phrases which triggered joviality. Think up your own to connect with your title and jot it down.

Then see if you can envisage how you might move from the amber situation back into consolidated green. If you feel that the client is already in red before you start, try and imagine what might have led to the situation in the first place. Track back to what happened before – remember the saucepan lid for Jack.

How would you use your biographical knowledge to flip the client from red to green?

Now picture yourself in that situation and work out how you would distract them from the past context in order to orientate them towards a present-day activity that they would readily accept.

A good example of a carer who was able to resolve a drastic problem by identifying a simple contextual explanation was Jennifer. She was baffled when her husband Jason insisted on leaving the house every evening just as they settled down to watch the six o'clock news. It was the one time of the day when she hoped to relax for a few minutes and catch up with the bigger-picture news. At that very point Jason would leap up, become extremely agitated, rattle the curtains and insist on leaving the house.

Penny asked Jennifer to write an exact account of the saga when it next happened. It turned out that Jason's chair was opposite the window and that they lived in a house that looked directly onto the street where many cars were parked. They had moved only two years before from a house in the country and Jason had always been most particular about any car being put away in the garage at night. As soon as he caught sight of cars outside the window in the street he became very agitated, wondering whether they were burglars or what. Once Jennifer understood where the anxiety was coming from and what Jason was trying to do, she worked on the above exercise and quickly came up with the solution. Before she turned on the TV she would point out the cars to Jason and say, 'They're so grateful to be able to park there – they'll be gone later on. Let's draw the curtains . . .' Jason immediately took charge of drawing the curtains.

The Red-to-Green exercise may take you some time but at the end of it, hopefully, you can see that agreeing and never interrupting are going to oil the wheels of your dealings with the client. Hopefully, also, you can see that it is possible to recover from disastrous red scenarios as well.

However, even when put together with what you have learned in the previous two chapters, there is still a great deal more you need to know before you are ready to deliver 24-hour wraparound care. The golden nugget at the heart of SPECAL is called the Primary Theme, explained in the next chapter.

TROUBLESHOOTING

'My mother has apparently adjusted to living in a care home, while still looking forward to going home when she is better. She recently became convinced that one of her family had died. How should I advise her professional carers to respond?'

Ask the carers to show polite interest whenever your mother makes this comment. They might perhaps say, 'Oh, really. Such an interesting person.' Ask them to jot down any follow-on remark that your mother then makes. She may agree, or disagree, or just drop the subject altogether. Tell the staff that you are interested in gathering more information about the whole topic, without actually asking any questions: who the family member is, what your mother knows about the circumstances of the death, whether she really minds, and what, if anything, she feels she should be doing about the situation. As the carers pick up more information from your mother, you will be able to use this to develop a conversational loop when she is feeling distressed about the situation.

THE RED-TO-GREEN LOOP

1. Validate the client – get alongside them, become a member of their club, join them where they are.

2. Analyse the biographical context of their concerns and use this information to flip from red to green.

3. Distract from biographical context to orientate them back into present-day activity. Choose a conversational ball from the client's collection, which you now have at your end of the court, as you play your way together through another routine activity of daily life.

CHAPTER SEVEN

The Primary Theme

In the stories from Part One many of the clients were enabled to have well-being by experiencing an aspect of their past as the present. Penny Garner's mother, Dorothy, often assumed that she was at an airport waiting to take a plane. Alice tended to assume rooms full of people were a Bridge Club as soon as she spotted a table with a crushed-velvet cloth. With Nellie the context for a meaningful existence was gardening, so her husband Richard's strategic placing of secateurs around the house enabled contented coexistence to replace dangerous acrimony.

In each case, by allowing and supporting the client's area of expertise and previously established world, SPECAL made them a present of this aspect of their past. This is not a matter of planting memories or encouraging delusions. It simply entails allowing the client to plug into long-term memories of real events that occurred in the past and forming links between them and the present moment. Past experience actually comes to be a great deal of their present; the past makes sense of the present.

SPECAL employs the term Primary Theme to denote the systematic use of photographs from long ago to create a context for the client through most of the present day. It is the royal road to dementia well-being and the most critical single technique for wraparound care. It enables the person to live much of their waking life in their favourite psychological place, an activity or interest that they have always loved, one that brings them alive, that promotes their feeling of self-worth. However, it is additionally benign because it protects against the greatest threat to their mental health, realising that they have not stored a recent event or information. So long as the client is absorbed in their theme there is no danger that they will be asking questions about who they are, who the people around them are, or what has happened to their memory.

It is very possible that you have already found the Primary Theme in one of the three favourite topics you identified for use as balls for verbal ping-pong. The theme can be almost anything at all, from architecture to bird watching to grumbling to jungle warfare. Once established, it provides the narrative out of which the day is constructed, largely replacing the awareness of the ever-changing present time, place and social context by which people without dementia organise themselves. As the illness gradually progresses it provides the basis for delivering 24-hour care in which no new photographs are needed and the client is wholly protected from the extreme peril of a red blank.

Although the theme is primary, other areas of significant interest can be connected to it. For example, if the theme is crosswords, it's always possible to find a way to link it to the most seemingly unrelated other themes from the past, like cooking or travel. So do not worry: in settling on a single Primary Theme you will not be ruling out visits to all other activities and interests as psychological places – in fact, you will be able to travel far and wide from this base. Advantageously, from your standpoint, the theme is also linked to the practical tasks of everyday life, enabling the client to go to the loo, put on or take off their clothes, eat and sleep. They are more than happy to do these when embedded in a context that is familiar and pleasurable to them (for example, 'You might want to have a bite to eat/have a nap/go to the loo before tackling the crossword . . .'). On top of that – and very happily for the client – the theme stimulates the opposite of the ghostly, pale-faced, empty death-mask expression that comes from feeling powerless and rudderless, so commonly the case for people with dementia not in SPECALCARE. Instead, they are calmly immersed in a pleasurable pursuit – the theme.

DOROTHY'S PRIMARY THEME

Like all other carers, Penny was learning on the hoof with Dorothy. Burford, let alone SPECAL, lay in the future. With her father Sam using common sense and Penny still learning, Dorothy's many interests and enthusiasms fell by the wayside one by one. If Penny had known then what she knows now, for example, Dorothy could have continued to play Bridge. Not as she had done in the past, as an international player, of course not. But with the help of her friends, suitably SPECALed, she could have continued to enjoy the social game and made sense of much of her life using its argot. The same goes for her interest in golf, which also went by the board. There are several other pastimes she could have 'played at' very happily, from the start of dementia to the end of her life. But as it was, the Primary Theme which Dorothy handed to Penny was 'Heathrow'. The thread of memories associated with it enabled Penny to sustain Dorothy's capacity to make sense of her life.

The first time Penny encountered Dorothy's airport theme

came as a considerable surprise. They were sitting in a crowded waiting room when out of the blue Dorothy said, 'Has our flight been called yet?' Penny was mystified and played for time, 'Er . . . not sure,' and, clutching her handbag and looking around anxiously her mother replied, 'We don't want to miss it – where's our luggage?' She tapped her neighbour's shoulder politely, 'Excuse me, is that your luggage?' pointing to their shopping bag. Penny pulled herself together and said, 'All our luggage is checked in. We've only got our handbags, everything else is checked in.' 'Oh, good,' said Dorothy cheerfully, and settled back.

From that epiphany onwards, Penny realised it was always a possibility that any crowded environment or waiting of any sort, turned into Heathrow when seen through Dorothy's eyes. Penny needed to be wherever Dorothy was, and accepting the Heathrow theme was the quickest and easiest way of achieving it in a wide variety of psychosocial settings.

An Aladdin's cave of possibilities opened up. Penny learned to play ping-pong using one or another travelling ball and it was easy to weave in the other parts of daily life. Almost whatever they were doing, they were waiting to go to the next place, which would be even more exciting than the last. It was interesting how much of one's life is spent waiting for the next thing to happen. The Heathrow scenario provided a rational and useful match, more or less, for many situations, be that a doctor's waiting room, a bus queue or a supermarket checkout. Dorothy would murmur something, quite casually, either about the flight being delayed, or passport control being rather slow, or the duty-free area being rather busy. Penny carefully noted her mother's use of language and fed it into their conversation, establishing a safe lexicon of familiar phrases. 'Let's form an orderly queue' was helpful for signalling a visit to the loo.

'Let's weigh it and see' came to mean 'let's wait and see'. They had their own code.

Dorothy had not lost her reason, merely the recent information as to what she and Penny had been doing moments before. She had no means of 'knowing' (in the way Penny 'knew') what exactly they were doing now. By Penny just smiling back and nodding in agreement, they could chat away about something else interesting to them both in order to while away the waiting moments. Dorothy would enter into the conversation (which obviously Penny made sure was about something well known to them from the past), and so they would wait, probably considerably less bored than everyone else waiting with them.

The only problem was making sure that reality kicked in at the right time, and that was definitely down to Penny, not Dorothy. On a need-to-know basis Dorothy needed to know about actual reality (doctor's surgery) only at the moment when an actual physical transition from one environment (waiting room) to another (consulting room) was absolutely imminent. Then she needed cues from Penny. Timing was crucial, and, rather like with a toddler, it paid to make special arrangements out of earshot of Dorothy, to ensure that Penny knew what their timing was likely to be.

Penny was the only one who knew what sense Dorothy was making and what sense they were both going to have to make in a moment's time. How could Dorothy prepare for a doctor's appointment when she was still waiting for her flight to be called? The context of the surgery had to be subtly introduced only when the doctor's receptionist told them to go into the consulting room. Penny soon learned in these situations that if she gave the information too early and then they had to wait longer, Dorothy would become anxious. It was evident in her face and general demeanour, her expression moving from cheerful to clouded. Her eyes would almost glaze over as she began to 'think' and try to reason out some mixed messages that didn't quite add up. Doctors became muddled with airports and this could only be bad news on a major scale.

There had been a particularly disturbing episode in Dorothy's life many years before. She had been going to take a flight to London but never boarded because she found the check-in clerk so rude and unhelpful. Returning to her hotel, she turned on the television to be confronted with horrendous pictures of what had occurred on the flight she should have been on: the jet had crash landed shortly after take-off, killing everyone on board. The connection between doctors and airports was not one Penny wished Dorothy to make.

Penny learned over and over again that it was disturbing to Dorothy to interfere with the sense she was making (the context for what she was seeing in front of her eyes) unless action to back up the new information was provided immediately. It was no good taking away one context – which was supported for Dorothy by various props and cues she had picked up for herself from the environment – before being able to provide her with another acceptable alternative context, complete with new props and cues to fit. It reminded Penny of the futility of trying to take something out of a small child's hands without first offering them some sort of replacement to hold their attention. When she got it wrong for Dorothy, she had turned out a light without making sure that another one was lit somewhere else to help show the way.

The Heathrow theme gave Penny freedom. She found she could easily leave Dorothy for a few moments by saying something along the lines of, 'I suggest you stay here and look after our hand-bags, I'll just go and check how they're doing.' Penny didn't find she had to talk about departure boards necessarily herself, but just fit the information that she gave to what Dorothy could accept. The language served them both well. Dorothy would happily remain in her seat, taking care of both their handbags (hand luggage to her), while Penny went off to ask the receptionist where they were in the queue. On being told, let's say, that there were two more patients in front of them, Penny would return to explain that it would be a bit more time yet. If Dorothy mentioned something about the flight being a bit late, Penny would agree, probably murmuring along the lines of 'Oh well, everything for the best.' Then when the second patient had gone in, Penny would imperceptibly change gear and start inserting the odd cue to prepare Dorothy for the forthcoming move from A to B.

She learned to do this by continuing to chat quite normally, but now introducing some new information in the form of 'It's our turn next . . . we'd better get ready to move, thank goodness *the doctor's* nearly ready to see us.' She learned to say this in a way that suggested they had been discussing waiting for the doctor many times in the past half hour, rather than living in the Heathrow scenario. She found that provided she gave out the information in a suitably matter-of-fact way, with no hint of it being brand-new information that had not been available before, Dorothy accepted the change of context, even though she was mildly puzzled by it. Surprised comprehension followed immediately if the call from the receptionist happened on cue. More likely than not, Dorothy would rise to her feet saying 'Good gracious, are we at the surgery? I had no idea.'

The open cheerfulness with which Dorothy expressed her perceptions meant that Penny learned fast. She discovered that puzzlement is not the same as deep anxiety. She could sense that Dorothy was saying to herself something like 'Oh, is *that* what they're doing! I had no idea! Goodness me, my memory really is getting very unreliable these days! Lucky you're here to remind me what I'm meant to be doing!' It was vital that Penny said 'we' are going and referred to 'our' appointment with the doctor. It was also important for Penny to match gestures to the words, and not rely on words alone, always reflecting Dorothy's own words and gestures, whenever possible.

On coming out of the doctor's, the best plan was to provide Dorothy with chat that inferred that they had had a really good time, without actually identifying in what way. There was no way Penny could know for sure whether Dorothy had stored what had just happened. Penny supplied general prattle, 'Well, that was all jolly good. Now I think we deserve a nice cup of tea.' Occasionally, Dorothy would mention something connected with the visit to the surgery, in which case Penny would follow that line and provide any necessary information, but that hardly ever happened. More often than not, just the knowledge that they had done something jolly together would do. Once out of the surgery it was usually as if it had not existed. In a curious way, life became extremely pleasant and quite intriguing, even exciting, because Penny never knew where they were going next.

The wraparound care which Dorothy's Heathrow theme conferred became the template for the rest of Penny's work. The Primary Theme, particular to each client, can provide total protection through access to an authentic identity in time and space. There has not been a single occasion during all the twenty years at Burford when it hasn't worked. Of course, the language and 'contexts' have been hugely varied, so that, among the hundreds of clients Penny has helped, no two themes have been exactly the same.

HOW TO IDENTIFY YOUR CLIENT'S PRIMARY THEME

In Dorothy's case, the client presented the Primary Theme already packaged up. While it may be as simple as that for you, more commonly a certain amount of forensic work is required.

In reading about Dorothy you may have found yourself suddenly reappraising seemingly incomprehensible, negligible or downright mad comments made by your client that up until now you have just ignored as meaningless static thrown up by haywire mental malfunctions caused by the illness. If you are already beginning to look afresh at previously meaningless behaviour, the Primary Theme that you need may already be sitting there before you. Once you reappraise the apparently inconsequential or rather alarming words or behaviour produced by the client, you may realise they make perfect sense when understood as coming from old pages of the album. The SPOT method, as described in Chapter 5, will help you make these connections.

Reappraise the questions and acceptable answers you noted down in that chapter, along with the topics found for verbal ping-pong in Chapter 4. You may find there was something that makes perfect sense when put in the context of the client's personal history. Perhaps the client is eternally asking where their handbag is or where Alan has gone or perhaps it is something that seems to make no sense at all, like why the moon is out in the day or why the fish are leaping about. In the vast majority of cases, once you know that these seemingly odd comments are coming from old pages, you can quickly relate them to the client's biographical history, using verbal ping-pong. For instance, there might be constant references to fish. Is this word always used as a noun (the animal) or sometimes as a verb (the sport) or even as an adjective, fishy? Are they talking about a time they went fishing or have they got a particular catch in mind? You need to see it as a game, becoming Sherlock Holmes and Sigmund Freud rolled up into one. Perhaps there are other quite different connotations – a bit fishy, a big fish (in a small pond), fishing for information, fish on Fridays, fish and chips, fish around, chip around, and who knows what you will find this all means to the client. As Sherlock Freud use your knowledge of what rings the client's bell to find out if this is the one for them. You need a pen and paper for what follows.

First of all, write down the client's interests, enthusiasms, achievements and hobbies during their life. Give your imagination free rein and let your mind float freely over the client's history, as far back as you like. Think of what may have been their 'finest hour'. Include interests that they do not necessarily still pursue – in fact, pay particular attention to ones that may have been most important several decades ago. For instance, Tina wrote down for her husband 'James Bond movies', 'darts', 'the beach in Devon', 'wine' and 'doing the pools'; in Tina's husband's case, darts eventually turned out to be the Primary Theme.

With your list of potential themes before you, a number of questions will most likely arise. Some carers wonder how they can be confident that these themes are truly what their client would feel are their main interests or enthusiasms. To put the boot on the other foot, imagine that you had dementia and further suppose either that your (pre-dementia) client was your carer or that someone else close to you was. If they were asked what your favourite pastimes, passions, interests had been or are, would they know? It's a jolly important question because they are about to choose one of these as the basis of your 24-hour wraparound care. In fact, reassuringly, the answer is most likely to be yes, the client or other carer would know. But in picking one out you would want them to take a fair amount of trouble so it is worth asking at least two other people who have been or currently are intimate with the client to make a list as well.

Once you have obtained the full list, write each one down on a separate line. The next thing is to put them in order, in terms of their feasibility as the Primary Theme. We will come in a moment to practical steps you can take to test them out, but for the time being, evaluate each one's suitability according to the following criteria:

- It should relate to long-term memories, so there should be a large number of photographs of the theme in the pre-dementia section of the client's album. Preferably, it is an interest or pastime that was most alive for the client many years ago, perhaps in their twenties or thirties, or even younger.

- It should be primarily associated with green, something that they enjoyed, which made them feel good: happy memories. That does not mean it will have had no disappointments associated with it. A man may have loved playing darts but there will have been occasions when he lost or played badly. That does not matter in itself, because the method will support his happy associations and gives you tools to convert the disappointments into hope for the future. If there is an associated red lurking in the shrubbery, you will be well placed to handle it by employing the Red-to-Green method described in Chapter 6.

- It should be something the client has pursued independently of you, even if you sometimes shared it. This is because they must have a strong sense of ownership and expertise within the theme. It is important that they do not associate you with similar expertise, as they will then lose that crucial sense of confidence that a fully owned Primary Theme can bring. It must be theirs and theirs alone. If the theme is doing crosswords exclusively with you, and if you are also a dab hand at them, it will not be so easy to make it into a fount of agency and self-esteem for them, and you should continue to look for something else.

- There needs to be a phrase to connote this theme *which is used by and generated by the client*. It needs to be something from their own personal, intimate lexicon, filled with resonances associated with those precise words. Hence, in the case of the carer Tina and her husband's darts, mentioned above, on closer inspection it emerged that he used the word 'arrows' and darts is only Tina's way of denoting it. So his Primary Theme was denoted as arrows, not darts, an important distinction in terms of its coming alive for him as a context for his life. This specificity of language becomes ever more essential as the illness progresses, so that merely saying the words will reassure the client – as soon as they know what is going on is related to 'arrows', 'Bridge', 'doing crosswords', 'waiting at the airport' or whatever, they can find meaning, coherence and peace.

- There needs to be a gesture to connote this theme and it is likely to have been originally generated by the client. It may be a sideways arm movement as if throwing a rugby ball, or a little finger movement as if inserting a jigsaw piece, or it could be just a minor flick of the head or a wink. Tina played conversational ping-pong several times before deciding that the best gesture was the raised right arm, as if about to throw the dart, an action that her client demonstrated. To begin with the gesture will be used sparingly but as the dementia gathers momentum the gesture will apply in an increasing number of contexts relating to daily life. Eventually, it can be used by anyone, communicating that they are part of this theme, that this is the psychological place where they are, the context. It becomes the reason why anxious questioning can be laid safely to rest.

For example, Jim's Primary Theme was swimming. He had trained professionally, demonstrating various strokes to Penny, and she did her best to imitate his style. One day he picked on her crawl: 'Not like that!' he said firmly, 'Like this!' He illustrated the perfect crawl stroke, which needless to say she never got completely right. They continued to talk about all sorts of things over the weeks and months, but the perfect crawl stroke kept coming up. Years later, when Penny went to see Jim in the nursing home, she had only to start the gesture of the crawl and Jim would smile and say knowingly, 'Not like that! Like this!' His whole world of expertise, of being in control, of having fun, was all tied up in that single gesture which had been repeated so often that it had become an important anchor in his life.

Using these criteria, pick out three themes from your list and put them in order: 1, 2, 3. Now you are nearly ready to start testing out which is best. You will have intimations, and they are probably right, but the only way to find out for sure is trial and error, using SPOT.

Divide three pages in your notebook down the middle. Write the first theme at the top of one page and down the left-hand side, list specific phrases for different aspects of the theme to use with the client. Suppose the theme was 'cooking'. For the phrases you might write 'Sunday lunch – the best in the world is at home', 'the fish and chips down the road', 'breakfast is the most important meal in the day' and so on. You can then spend a day introducing cooking whenever possible, and give a score from 1 to 10 evaluating how much well-being each of the different comments brings. On subsequent days, do the same with the remaining two themes. So long as you keep a close eye on the reactions you get to the different themes overall and to the specific words with which you prompt them, you should get a reasonable idea of how much well-being the different old pages provide.

In Chapter 2 I described Penny's early work at Burford and her use of Irish reels when she first started communicating with Paddy. For some time Penny assumed that reels would be his theme, or if not that, something Irish at least. But Paddy was a baker by trade and an excellent one at that. Primarily he was a master baker who could reel, rather than a reeler who could bake. For most of the time, discussion of Ireland, its landscape and its sports (including more often than not, reeling, which led to fishing) took the front stage, but the all-important background scenery that provided confidence to Paddy was his position as a baker. Master baking was the umbrella under which so many other subsidiary topics resided. This theme, with its associated links, became a successful means for making sense of every other part of Paddy's life when at the hospital – arriving, eating and drinking, going to the bathroom, getting dressed or undressed, staying the night, leaving.

It is really important to take things slowly and to beware of putting the client under pressure in relation to the selected Primary Theme. Robert had been keen on aeroplanes since a boy and was in the RAF during the war when he met his wife in the WAAF. He was particularly fascinated and excited by night flying, which he had done a lot of during the war. He also had an interest in birds and was very knowledgeable about them. Penny found it easy to move between planes and birds with the gesture of fingers splayed, swooping through the air in front of her. She got quite good at switching themes by saying 'Oh that looks like a bird, or maybe it's a plane.' He'd say 'Ah now, planes', and off he would go. He also had cricket as a theme. So many of his family had played for the county team, seven or eight playing at one time, that it was known locally as Smithshire rather than its real name. In short, he was multi-talented and there were a lot of well-being-conferring interests.

In the end, Penny went for night flying as the Primary Theme, partly because there was a book he had with that title, written by a friend of his and in which he was mentioned by name, including photographs. Penny had only to point at the book, mention the title and he was away. One day Penny gave the book to a helper at Burford, having explained its significance, leaving her to get on with it. Unfortunately, the assistant plunged in with another aeroplane-related book she had found with some writing and pictures of the nearby air base, Brize Norton. She asked Robert a direct question about the air base, requiring considerable detail of Robert, and he went from amber to red very quickly indeed. The next day his wife fed back that he felt he had been tested recently and had failed. He had no clear recollection of where and when the test had taken place, just that he had a feeling of fear and failure. He then said categorically that he didn't want to talk about night flying because it was too worrying. A week later, his wife reported that he was now having nightmares around a ghastly incident towards the end of the war in which friends had died in their planes and it had left him feeling he should not have survived.

Night flying was fitting the bill perfectly until the helper pressed far too many buttons too fast, causing him to be overwhelmed. The theme had to be abandoned and another one found. Fortunately, Penny was able to switch to birds. She had heard on Radio 4 of a competition to find the most birds in your backyard and sent off for details of how to enter. She invited Robert to help them win the competition the next time he came and to bring his binoculars. Together they began a list of birds seen from the Day Unit window and soon Robert was happily peering out into the garden through them. He spotted a robin and then a crow, and so they moved on. After a considerable passage of time Robert began to talk about aeroplanes again but never to the extent that he had done right at the start.

PROPS AS CUES AND TRIGGERS OF THE PRIMARY THEME

As aficionados of the Orson Welles film *Citizen Kane* will know, it opens with a newspaper magnate lying on his deathbed uttering the word 'rosebud'. It ends with us learning that the word was painted on a sled that Kane was riding as a child the day his mother sent him away. The sled is a token of the only time in his life when he was truly happy, united with his mother and wanting for nothing, emotionally. In SPECAL terms, the sled is a prop, something that reminds the client of their Primary Theme, the word 'rosebud' is all that is needed to trigger or cue it. If you were Charles Foster Kane's carer, you would also develop a gesture denoting rosebud, perhaps a cupping of the hands to indicate the petals in a flower.

We need a prop, a physical object, and verbal and gestural cues for your client's theme. Indeed, you might like to imagine yourself writing a Citizen Kane-style biography of your client's life: what would be the sled and the rosebud in their case? Unfortunately, the answer is unlikely to immediately spring to mind and you will probably have to work to establish it.

The great value of props and cues to the client is that they convey a wealth of meaning that would take many words to express. However, they need to be very few indeed, be very carefully chosen and relate directly to the Primary Theme. Like all the efforts to explore what will work best, you need to start with plenty and then whittle them down, using SPOT to see which carry the strongest message to the client.

IDENTIFYING PHYSICAL PROPS WHICH CUE THE PRIMARY THEME

There will already be innumerable props in your client's life that you can list – their newspaper crossword, pipe, handbag, glasses – a whole collection of artefacts the client regards as important, some of them of practical assistance, some for entertainment. You may find that you can work backwards from these props in choosing your theme. For example, a carer realised that her husband's theme was golf, by noticing that when he was watching golf on TV he used the remote control as a prop for it. The remote and the golf had become almost interchangeable, so she gradually inferred that when he was holding the remote or looking at it, golf was on his mind. More commonly, though, you need to work from the theme to the prop.

If you write the theme down at the top of a notebook page, allow your mind to float freely in considering what the props might be. For example, one carer had identified 'travel' as his wife's theme. As potential props, he came up with 'travel diaries' (she kept them), 'photos of trips', 'passport', 'brochures', 'luggage labels' and 'suitcase'. As always, the way to identify what worked best was to SPOT. However, in advising this carer, Penny made some provisos.

While actual photographs can provide a useful starting point for uncovering information, they will eventually need phasing out as they tend to be far from helpful as time goes by. Photographs require a great deal of 'now let me think' from the client and that is exactly what we are aiming ultimately to avoid. A client may find an actual photograph sends them to amber or red because they have a sense that they ought to know the who, where, when or why of the scene, yet part or all of it is missing.

The second proviso is simple. When Penny settled Dorothy into her excellent nursing home, The Professor said 'Make sure she has nothing with her that she or you would care about if it was lost.' The reason is the practical fact that the client is liable to leave objects anywhere or everywhere. Props, therefore, need to be items that can easily be replicated. You will need many versions of each. The ultimate goal is to whittle them down to a single object. When the dementia is more advanced that's all that will be needed, along with a few key words and gestures, to connote the theme – another reason to have something that can be replicated easily.

For example, Carl loved doing crosswords. He was very good at them and would sit for a long time on his own, with the dictionary at his side. What he also needed was a pencil with a rubber on the end, as did anyone else who sat beside him. Real crossword enthusiasts, in Carl's view, used a pencil with a rubber on the end. 'That's a proper pencil,' he would say approvingly, as his neighbour produced one. It was important to be a member of the 'we've got proper pencils' club when engaging with Carl. For Robert, the erstwhile night flyer turned birdwatcher, binoculars became his bird watching prop. A great advantage of these was that in the early stages it was easy to have several pairs lying around the house. In the later stages, it only required the binocular case in order to cue him into the theme. It was the same with Nellie's secateurs, described in Chapter 3.

At least in the early stages, you will have more than one prop. It often takes time for the main one to emerge, ultimately selected by the client's reaction. You will need one prop that travels easily, for going to the shops or trips to the doctor. As with all other aspects of SPECALCARE, that is your lodestar: how words, actions and key objects around the client make them feel, with maximum sense of identity and resultant well-being as the goal.

The Shangri La of well-being is called the Moment of Care. By this, Penny means that the client is totally absorbed with what is going on, enlivened, excited or quietly contented, in the best possible place. A Moment of Care may last seconds or hours or days. Apart from the happiness of it as a state, it is doubly beneficial because the client is at nil risk of a red. All anxious questioning is suspended and the person is operating on autopilot, their attention held in the same way as a small child at the pantomime, caught up in the magnetic magic of the moment.

IDENTIFYING KEY WORDS AND GESTURES
TRIGGERING THE THEME

While establishing props you can also keep a close eye out for both words and gestures that cue the theme. Indeed, these may cue in the prop (thereby cueing in the theme). Just saying the word for the prop may eventually be sufficient without having to physically produce it – saying 'binoculars' or 'binocular case' could sometimes have the same effect as actually having them for Robert. Likewise, holding both hands up to the eyes with the fingers curled and peering through them in an imitation of someone looking through binoculars could take Robert instantly down the chain of connections from gesture of binoculars to binoculars to bird watching.

To establish key words, start on a new page of your notebook with the theme written at the top and jot down the ones that are used by the client in connection with the theme. During the course of a day, try to score which of the words or phrases are most often used. It's critical not to impose your own vocabulary. As noted in the example above, the carer who picked darts as the name of her husband's theme was using the wrong word. A mention of arrows almost literally picked him up. A mention of darts was likely to be ignored.

Using this method you should create a small lexicon of words or phrases that strongly engage the client in a positive way and connote the theme to them. Taking one day, try the different words out and score how much success they achieve out of 10 in promoting conversation of some sort about the theme.

Now follow the same procedure with gestures. In this case, the client will have a smaller number of potential ones, or there may be none at present. Using your imagination, consider what gestures you would use in a game of charades to convey that theme to your client.

If it is 'doing the crossword', for example, you might act out someone with a pen looking down at a small square with a puzzled look on their face, counting off letters on their fingers. Once you have a list of potential gestures, as with the key words, over the course of a day give them a score out of 10 as to which is most effective in stimulating recognition of the theme. Start introducing it where you can, to reinforce what you are saying. Once you have found something that works, then repeat it as much as possible. You will soon know if you are overdoing it because the client will point it out. If this happens, it's time for something along the lines of 'Silly me. I seem to be turning into a windmill. Do forgive my waving arms!'

HOW THE PRIMARY THEME ACHIEVES
WRAPAROUND CARE

Once you have got the Primary Theme up and running, complete with props, key words and gestures, you will have the basis for 24-hour wraparound care that provides well-being for the rest of the client's life. If done successfully, it really does enclose the client in a chain of Moments of Care. Crucially, when all the elements have been put in place, it can be delivered by almost anyone who is willing to learn and it is simple. Although it may not seem like this right now, when you have got the Primary Theme working you will see that your main job as a SPECAL carer is to develop a programme of care so that you can start to teach others to deliver it as well as yourself.

Eventually, it will be possible for the client to enter a nursing home happily, and ultimately you will only need to visit them once a week. By this time all the information you have gathered and, importantly, used on a daily basis, will have been distilled into a single piece of paper, which Penny calls the client's SPECAL Passport. Before you can write it, there are two crucial, if subsidiary, additional tools which you need to identify: the Health Theme and the Explanations, outlined in the succeeding two chapters.

The Health Theme offers an essential acceptable context within which the client is able to accept help from other people without loss of dignity and without any unnecessary awareness of their dementia. Without this the care of the client would become impossible to manage.

TROUBLESHOOTING

'My husband has always had a great number of interests, and his dementia isn't very far advanced, so should I wait for things to move on a bit before I decide on the Primary Theme?'

The Primary Theme needs selecting as soon as possible after diagnosis, so you certainly should not delay making your choice. The dementia is far more advanced than you realise. If you were asking your question at Burford, Penny would open up a metronome which sits on her desk, and talk about the tick-tock of the dementia clock and the need for action, not delay. Until you have identified the Primary Theme and given it a name, you cannot make any progress with anything else to do with wraparound care.

'I am down to the last two on my list of Primary Themes, and am getting quite stressed about deciding which one to choose. Surely there's room for more than one?'

Having more than one Primary Theme is the equivalent of having none. It is as if you are asking someone to talk half in one language and half in another, while you juggle two dictionaries on your lap trying to decide which one to look at as they progress through their sentence. A single Primary Theme is crucially and urgently required.

You will become less stressed if you imagine that you are playing a game of Desert Island Discs, but with a choice of Primary Theme for your client instead of a favourite piece of music. You have been allowed to talk about eight choices, but now, at the end of the programme, it is time to select *the* one favourite. You choose the one which is the most powerful in terms of feelings, and it becomes the encapsulation and distillation of all the rest. You have not lost the experience of the other seven but you will only have room for one in your survival pack.

'I don't want to limit myself to just one topic when I visit my mother, because we talk about such a rich variety of things whenever we meet.'

It is really important that you continue to visit and talk in the same way with your mother as you always have, and that the selection of the Primary Theme doesn't herald any immediate change. However, your observational skills will be heightened when you hold a focus of your mother as an expert in one particular area, and you start listening out for ways in which connections with words, phrases and gesture might be made. One carer recently spent a whole workshop trying to come to terms with the final selection of Primary Theme for her mother. Eventually, and extremely reluctantly, she agreed to 'go with' the selection of 'Potato Marketing Board Demonstrator' which was one of three at the top of her list, although she was far from convinced that she had made a wise choice. Penny persuaded her that any choice would be better than no choice, and that she should not leave the workshop without a final decision – she had to grow up!

The following week Penny heard via e-mail that the carer had gathered up at least three new useful quotes from her mother, had identified an excellent gesture of the way baking potatoes should be pricked, and had already used the theme in relation to achieving various practical tasks which had been causing great difficulty. There had been no change to the rich variety of conversational routines with her mother, but these were now being fitted into a cohesive pattern which clearly worked. The carer reported that she felt amazingly positive about the progress she had made once the Primary Theme was named and used at home and had lost nothing in the process.

TO IDENTIFY AND USE A PRIMARY THEME

1. Make a long list of areas of past interest for your client. Include as much as possible under the following headings:
   - They loved doing it
   - They could do it without effortful thinking
   - They used to do it quite a bit of the time
   - They used to talk about it

2. Decide which are the top three, scored by your view of:
   - how early in life the interest first arose
     plus
   - the ease of association with a sense of achievement for the client
     plus
   - the likelihood that the client would have been prepared to engage with people with a similar interest, in the past

3. Choose just one area of client interest and create a title phrase, starting with the word 'Expert', to convey status to your client. Don't worry that you may have got the 'wrong one'. You can make any of them work – you just have to get on and choose one.

4. From now on, think of your client primarily as an expert in this field, and think of everyone else (including yourself) as being keen to pick up handy tips from the client.

5. Remember that all other interests on your original list can be linked in, not lost, through the creation of the Primary Theme.

6. Remember to treat the Primary Theme with great respect for the owner of it – it is the client's topic, not your own!

7. Brush up your own knowledge around the Primary Theme by reading about it or talking to other people. You need to use this information to become more expert at pitching your need for help at the right level for the client.

8. List vocabulary associated with the Primary Theme.

9. Work out how to make easy connections between the Primary Theme vocabulary, other past pleasures and the routine activities of life today.

10. Learn to love repeating what works for the client.

11. SPOT which props work best for the client, and choose just one or two as crucial props to use on a repeated basis, every day.

12. Have the confidence to use repetition more rather than less. You will rarely, if ever, overstep the mark. Better by far to discover that you have overdone the degree of repetition (you can correct it so easily by using the 'Silly me' tool), than to err on the dangerously cautious side of common sense. Dementia is ticking along, and you need to keep up with it and use it as a positive resource.

CHAPTER EIGHT

The Health Theme

Alongside the Primary Theme, it is essential to have another theme from the old pages in the client's photograph album to help them to attend to practical day-to-day activities of ordinary life. Put bluntly, if your client is only immersed in the world of their bird watching or Heathrow airport lounge or rugby it can be hard to get them to eat, sleep and go to the loo. Moreover, you have to shift the emphasis from their reinforced sense of independent skill and prowess to a dignified need to accept help in a sensible way from another person. You have to identify acceptable reasons for various kinds of transitions between places, carers and social situations and you will only be able to do this when you have the twin to the Primary Theme in place: the Health Theme.

THE HEALTH THEME

The Primary Theme works wonders for the client's well-being by boosting their self-esteem and giving them a strong sense of agency and control. Quite often, you will be able to knit the Primary Theme into everyday life activities using the we-relationship, so that 'we' break off from playing Bridge for a spot of lunch or 'we' decide not to finish a crossword tonight so there will be some left to do tomorrow. But the Primary Theme is sometimes too effective at raising the client's self-esteem to the point where they imagine they need no help from anyone. You have boosted them so much that their ego has become over-inflated and you need a way to get them to come back down to earth before they float away altogether, like a helium balloon. It is one thing protecting them as far as you possibly can (never totally, but to a very large extent) from an awareness of their condition, and quite another to leave them unaware of the need for any help in any direction. All of us need help from time to time, but the person with dementia needs a lot. A reality check of some sort is required to enable them to overlap with the rest of the world.

If you attempt to convince them they cannot cope on their own but have no explanation of why, they will – not having lost the ability to reason – deduce their own explanation. This is extremely perilous because, as they leaf back through their album in search of factual information that makes sense of their incapacity, their dependence on others, they are almost bound to find it in the section recording their diagnosis. For most people these photographs are irredeemably red. So if there is no technique for switching out of the Primary Theme, the client may develop a sense of unfettered, unobstructed independence and sense of their own expertise, while living in a time warp. This has only one eventual outcome: they become entirely unmanageable, something they certainly would not want if they were able to analyse the situation. Enter the Health Theme.

This theme provides an acceptable reason for the client to become dependent on your advice again, to start listening to you rather than being the expert who is in control. This is not so much a reversal as a balance, to ensure equilibrium between the world of the client and everyone else. The Health Theme derives from the fact that all of us can accept the need to avoid illness and for convalescence. Since everyone (and especially older people) has had medical reasons at some point in their life for having to shut down and disconnect from their favourite occupations, if you identify the right one from your client's old pages and use their words to signal it, this will usually act as a brake.

SOME EXAMPLES

John was so deeply entrenched in a sense of well-being brought on by his Primary Theme that he refused to go to bed at all. He had been the manager of a munitions factory and felt that he had pretty well won the war single-handedly by inspiring ever greater results on the production line. He used to sit in the small reception area of the hospital, checking the staff in as they arrived for their shift. Even the hospital manager was prepared to be checked in by John, admonished for her late arrival, and would promise to make up for it at once. One evening John seemed to change gear and began to work absolutely flat out. Clearly the war was gathering momentum and he needed to match that with extra effort. He insisted a dying patient get out of their bed and get on with their job. There was no scope in John's schedule for employees taking a break and the nursing staff had huge problems that night as they struggled to care for patients appropriately. Penny Garner was summoned the next morning by the hospital manager and told that unless she could sort the problem out, dementia patients would no longer be admitted overnight and SPECAL was likely to become a thing of the past.

A quick search of the notes revealed that John had suffered from osteoporosis from well before the onset of dementia. Having studied John's own language when referring to his illness, 'osteoporosis' became 'this silly back', an ailment that even the most efficient munitions factory manager might agree needed attending to. Really, he must get some rest if only to ensure that he could get on with the job in the best possible way the next day. From then on, the nurses began tempering their use of the Primary Theme with John by this newly acquired Health Theme and it worked a treat. Henceforth, all clients coming into the hospital overnight had a Health Theme clearly established before being checked in. With both themes in place and carefully used, a balance between independence and acceptable dependency on others could be sustained around the clock.

For example, Tom had had dysentery while on active service in India. His treatment had been successful but he was always concerned that he should never get the illness again, so it was easy to press that button. Stan had a damaged elbow, brought about by a cricket ball. As it happened, cricket was also his Primary Theme, a happy confluence. Another client had long-standing diabetes that worked so well it led Penny to ask new carers in a half-hopeful way, 'I suppose your client doesn't suffer from diabetes, by any chance?' Flat feet, an out-of-alignment collarbone, prostate problems – you name it, Penny has had it on her books. Heart bypass, cancer of this, cancer of that – provided it pre-dates the dementia by as long as possible and had a satisfactory outcome from the client's perspective, it's the business.

WIDER USES OF THE HEALTH THEME

It turned out that the Health Theme's applications extended beyond situations where the Primary one had got out of control. Penny used Dorothy's in numerous situations where orientation to a present task was needed. For Dorothy, the choice of theme had been easy, having had a cancer scare well before dementia. She had been sent post-haste to the Royal Marsden where she remained for several days having fairly invasive tests. Luckily, the news was good and Dorothy was free to leave. She could not do so fast enough and they were soon having tea together on the train going home. She said she was the luckiest person alive and so much more fortunate than others in her ward who were staying on for difficult treatments. She marvelled at the way just a couple of words could spell out a desperate scenario or signal a complete return to normal life. 'I've got the *all-clear*,' she kept saying, 'I am the luckiest person alive.' Penny had what she needed, if ever she had to explain an assessment process to her. 'We've got the all-clear, and must keep it that way,' Penny would say, knowing that this was flagging up an old set of memories about being lucky and feeling grateful, a health encounter which had a good outcome.

Penny hardly ever had to use it in relation to health checks (there were none in the formal sense as her GP father Sam generally took charge of the family's ailments) but she did use it to manoeuvre through activities of daily life. One day Penny was hovering in Dorothy's room trying to help her change her clothes in order to go out in the evening. Dorothy said 'Why on earth can't I do all this for myself? Is there something wrong with me?' Penny knew exactly what Sam would have to say if Dorothy appeared in any way less than perfectly turned out. So Penny said, 'We've got the all-clear, and that's what really matters.' Dorothy immediately cheered up, looked brightly at her and said, 'I'm the luckiest person alive.' As she said this, Penny felt the same about herself, because she had managed to whisk off the problematic dress, which was on back to front, and was already well on the way to a much better look for Dorothy. Only the slightest encounter with the Health Theme was required, but it was a dusting of gold on an otherwise potentially nightmarish situation.

Over the years, Penny has found that most carers are able to use the Health Theme in daily management, as well as a check against an out-of-control Primary Theme. Usually, a GP appointment to investigate the client's memory problems is itself a horrendous problem when you try to explain it to the client. They may hotly deny there is anything wrong (while being painfully aware that there is) and things are very awkward for everyone, not least the doctor. If the carer confronts the client with evidence that their memory problems are evident to everyone, the client will add depression to their list of difficulties. But if framed as only a compulsory annual general health check, where medication is reviewed to make sure that dosage is the minimum required, it is much more acceptable. It makes sense for older people to look after their health, and the carer has no difficulty in using the we-relationship, insisting that both they and the client go and get checked.

During the Burford Hospital days, Penny introduced a generic Health Theme which applied to every client: 'got to keep ourselves up to date with the NHS requirements so we can get free treatment in our older age'. Linked to the particular Health Theme, the combined strength of the two is awesome. The explanation to the client by the carer has now become, 'We're going to the doctor to be checked out, not because there is something wrong with either of us but (quite the opposite) because we want to stay well. Also we're entitled to a review because of our age.' That sense of entitlement is great stuff for a client, who needs a sense of ownership about things more than most. Then again, the age bit is a cinch for the carer to talk about when they need to refer to anything remotely health- or dependency-related – authentic, quietly confident, matter-of-fact, we've just got-to-do-this-sensible-thing-together – just the sort of style SPECAL is promoting to the carer for just about everything. Penny finds that having this generic theme in place means that it can be introduced during fireside chats (part of verbal ping-pong, using SPOT), so that a special phrase – a mnemonic – can be established by the carer, using the client's own words. This phrase can then be used to explain not only doctor's appointments but also anything that needs promoting in terms of routine at home. 'We need to go to bed now, because of such and such.'

Penny has found that carers are able to establish predictable phrases, mostly along the lines of 'The doctor says we must [do whatever] . . .' or 'Dr X likes us to . . .' or 'we must listen to the quack and [do whatever] . . .' The phrase can be used by the carer to endorse actions at home, even tricky toileting ones, as they are being carried out – 'Dr X will be really pleased!' Just try it out yourself: you will see that if you develop this through ping-pong as part of your daily exchanges with the client it really works well. The doctor's imprimatur gives whatever is being considered a certain respectability, a gravitas, and importantly at the same time a sense of ownership by the client – as in 'my medical needs must be met, which I am entitled to because of my age'. In ping-pong terms this is a fascinating ball which can provide a long and meandering rally. Penny reports many versions of the following:

CARER: We're pretty good for our age really . . .

CLIENT: Well, I feel great. How old am I, anyway?

CARER: You're lucky, you look so young. It's hardly fair . . .

CLIENT: That's because I keep fit with rugger . . . now there's nothing like rugger for getting a bit of a sweat up . . . I remember the time when Bloggs was out on the wing, I was on his inside and he . . . and I . . .

Of course, using the generic or the Health Themes at home is one thing; it's quite another to visit an actual doctor. Penny has countless stories regaled to her by carers of difficult trips to a consultant or GP, or equally challenging visits by the community psychiatric nurse at home. All were trying to do their best and failing to do anything except exacerbate the situation. In some cases, there was a noticeable deterioration in client well-being at the time or afterwards, with the carer bearing the brunt back home.

Yet this could be avoided by an appropriate use of an individualised Health Theme, just ahead of the visit. The assessment visit (which is what it usually is) can be presented to the client in terms of how it needs to be perceived, as: a sensible, age-related health check. But crucially, that also calls for the professional concerned to be properly briefed. Unfortunately, many professionals have no idea of the huge damage that breaking the SPECAL three commandments can do. They are very prone to asking questions and to contradicting the basics of the Primary Theme. They need to understand that their visit is being viewed as part of a generic check up, not about dementia at all. They must allow the carer and the client to visit together as a single unit, to understand the 'we-relationship', so that client and carer are members of the 'we're having a nice visit to make sure we get everything that we're entitled to as we grow old gracefully' club. That's a far cry from the usual story.

In some cases, the potency of a Health Theme to protect against distress is astonishing. Mary's Primary Theme was 'Being part of a large family.' It was hard to identify a Health Theme for her because she had been so incredibly healthy all her life. Fortunately, she had had the odd problem with a toe now and then, and her Health Theme was therefore 'problem feet'. Her husband Paul was very good at the 'we' scenario and so visits to the doctor were relatively easy to present to Mary without flagging up dementia in any way. But two or three years after being diagnosed with dementia Mary developed a cough that turned out to be caused by a collapsed lung due to secondary cancer. The primary cancer had remained undetected until the secondaries were well into their stride. The cough worried Paul enough to have it investigated, although it worried Mary comparatively little, and she confined her attention to it to a 'cough-cough' phrase, rather similar to a tut-tut, every time she coughed. In between, she appeared to be unaware of any problem at all. Once the diagnosis was confirmed, the prognosis was sufficiently poor to indicate that Mary was likely to be requiring a good deal of nursing support in the almost immediate future. By now Mary was beginning to add to her 'cough-cough' statement that 'I really must get something done about that.' Paul, well versed in SPECAL techniques, adopted her phrases himself and so every time Mary coughed would say, 'cough-cough', to which Mary would respond, 'Yes, I must do something about it.' This gave Paul the consent he needed to echo this sentiment himself, using the 'we' approach, and pointed the way to the cough becoming a far more useful Health Theme than problem feet were ever likely to be.

From then on, visits to the oncologist were presented in the form of shopping trips, to cover the period from leaving the house to arriving in the hospital car park. Then, as they walked in and sat in the waiting area, the answer to Mary's question, 'What are we doing?' was 'Cough-cough . . . getting the cough sorted.' 'Oh!' Mary would say, 'That's all right then.' Because the cough was so frequent, and because the phrase used by everyone was Mary's phrase and was repeated each time, some of those cough statements became stored in Mary's memory. The oncologist was briefed that asking Mary about her breathing would not elicit any information from her, whereas a reference to a 'cough' would be likely to elicit at least agreement that she had a problem in that area.

Mary's story is uplifting because her experience of cancer – even when spread to three separate locations by the end – was largely limited to cough-cough, little more than a tut-tut in her life. The diagnosis of cancer was new information that she never stored. On a need-to-know basis it did not exist for her, beyond a validation of her own thought that she would do something about the cough in due course.

These examples show how helpful a Health Theme can be. So, the time has now come to identify your client's own theme.

IDENTIFYING YOUR CLIENT'S HEALTH THEME

To identify it you need to trawl the client's old pages and write down four or five occasions when they were not well, were dependent, or encountered health services and the doctor. In doing this, as much as possible try and recall the keywords the client would use to describe this incident. You are focusing entirely on the period well before the onset of dementia.

For example, one carer listed the following about his wife:

- 'Her parents' divorce in her early teens was the most tragic part of her life – worst moment. She ended up in therapy to sort things out.'

- 'She was fat as a child, entailing endless visits to doctors and specialists.'

- 'She had a breakdown after having kids.'

- 'She has immobile feet, I happen to think because she always wore those orthopaedic sandals. When I first knew her she had them on all the time. You have to crunch your toes up to keep them on your feet, clenched. Her toes do actually relax up after a while if she gets help. For most of our marriage she used to go to a reflexologist and it worked beautifully. The rest of her body relaxed, too.'

- 'She had her gall bladder out. She had a very bad patch with it, pain in the lead up to the operation, which was quite terrifying to me. She was lying around on the floor in agony. The worst thing was I bought the best surgeon in the world and he promised only a half inch cut but it was six inches, a terrible thing to have done to a woman.'

In helping the client to choose from this list, Penny reminded him that they were seeking a health problem that had a happy outcome but that could still require attention. Which would you choose? (That's right, only the foot problem fits this criterion.)

Another carer described the Health Theme candidates like this:

'As a child Charlie was delicate. The doctor, when he called, would say, "If you've sent for me, Charlie must be at home." He had mastoids as a child but the big problem has always been his ears. He always has been deaf. There is a phrase of his, he'll refer to himself, using irony, as handicapped: "Your attitude to the handicapped leaves a lot to be desired." I always say back "It's all my fault that you can't hear me."'

The deafness was the obvious candidate as Charlie's Health Theme. Penny's observation was that the carer should not be discouraged by the client's deafness or regard it as an impediment to SPECALCARE. The next step was to explore gesture associated with the deafness – those little signals which speak more loudly than words.

As always, once you have identified the most likely candidate for the Health Theme, use SPOT to check it out. If there is more than one possibility, write down each one on a separate sheet of paper. Then write the words or gestures the client uses in referring to that particular topic on the left-hand side of the paper. Once you have several phrases or gestures, over the course of a few days give scores of 1 to 10 over on the right-hand side of the paper to show how positively each one resonates with the client. Keep this up for a while and your list will soon tell you which theme is best and which key words or gestures are the best cues for it.

Having identified the Health Theme we are ready for the final set of tools: Explanations, which we will discuss in Chapter 9.

TROUBLESHOOTING

'My father has been well all his life. I can think of no time when he has been ill and he has never been in hospital. He just hasn't got a Health Theme.'

It is essential to select a Health Theme in order to avoid any direct, unnecessary and potentially catastrophic focus on dementia. Use the we-relationship as you play ping-pong with the topic of wishing to remain fit in the future and the best way of achieving this. You may uncover recollections from your father around the topic of his own parents having become less independent. His feelings and views about this could open the way to agreeing with you the importance of taking care of one's own health for the future. You need to find a phrase which he uses in this connection. One carer settled for 'Keeping fit and staying that way', which worked well for their client.

TO IDENTIFY THE HEALTH THEME

1. Make a list of any encounter you can think of between the client and health services in the past.
2. It needs to have had a positive outcome – not necessarily a cure but a satisfactory conclusion.
3. Choose the best.
4. Don't worry about how it links in, at this stage. Just choose one, give it a title, and move on.

CHAPTER NINE

Explanations

One of the commonest complaints – often the last straw – that carers make about their role is that they do not even get privacy in the bathroom. Their time is taken up with cooking, cleaning, shopping and domestic work, and sometimes with trying to keep the client from doing crazy or dangerous things, but on top of all that, the client is liable to follow them everywhere. Penny Garner has a simple solution. Weird though it may sound, she claims that you should never, ever leave the room, whether for a brief moment or a long time, without explaining to the client that you are going, and why. Rather, you need to develop an explanation for leaving and another explanation for your absence when gone. Both Explanations need to be completely acceptable and satisfying to the client, and then used again and again. The dementia will take care of the repetition, making it invisible. Endlessly duplicated, repeated like a parrot, the Explanations may eventually no longer need to be spoken, they merely require a gesture to convey the required message of serenity for the client. What bliss lies ahead for the carer: a peaceful, uninterrupted visit to the loo!

The reason it is so important not to leave the room without an explanation is that your departure could mean anything. You have to get inside your client's head to understand this. An unexplained departure potentially provokes some terrible questions: Where's she going? Is she going for half a day, all day? Is she going to see somebody I should know about? Severe panic can arise from this very simple thing. You are like an extra set of pages in their photograph album and if you leave inexplicably they know they are going to be left without information on today's page. It's terrifying. Basic information that you and I take for granted about what has just been going on moments before is denied them. As this situation repeats day after day, so the morass of non-existent information from previous weeks, months and years builds up. You have to understand that, whatever the appearances, the client is severely disabled. Penny never ceases to be amazed at the skill clients employ to cover up the problems. They are concealing 90 per cent of the stress and the strain; you only see the tip of the iceberg.

For example, a carer called Francis described how his wife sometimes goes off to their studio room to do jigsaws on her own. He would leave her in the sitting room and often find her in the studio when he arrived back. He asked Penny whether she did this to escape the pressure or because she is still confident enough to go off alone. Penny explained that she will almost certainly have got there via a series of unanswered questions drifting in and out of her mind. These questions will have been on amber and were sometimes prevented from turning to red by something in the environment which prompted her to head for the studio. She's got blanks or only fragments of recent photographs. 'Where's Francis?' she thinks, when left alone even for a few moments. She has no information on the page to tell her. She goes to look for him in the hall and shouts out 'Francis?' Referring again to today's pages, she thinks 'Well, there's not much here – no clues as to his whereabouts . . . now let me think . . .'

As she resumes her amber pondering, about to take a much closer look at her album and to begin leafing back, she looks around the room, catches sight of a jam jar with paintbrushes in it and makes a connection. She thinks 'Go to the studio; perhaps that's what I need to be doing.' When there, she sees a jigsaw and thinks 'Ah yes.' She settles into it, and is quickly absorbed. She has found a safe context, one where she only needs to look down to be reminded of what she has just been doing and this provides the clue to what she needs to do now – search for another jigsaw piece that fits. The level of absorption of a client once they are held by a familiar activity in this way is quite astounding. They are not 'thinking' in the sense of processing lots of facts, because they are on autopilot. The joy of a jigsaw puzzle to an enthusiast is that it is a compulsive activity that can trigger a state of sustained contemplation. It would make an ideal Primary Theme. In fact Francis had chosen dried flower arranging for his wife but Penny couldn't resist asking him whether he could find a jigsaw puzzle with a picture that fitted that theme. She also suggested finding a way of cueing in a trip to the studio *before* rather than after he left his wife alone, and finding a suitable explanation for his own departure once they were both in the studio. This would mean she would be left on a green that would stay green, rather than the Russian roulette game he was unwittingly playing when he left her on amber in the sitting room.

A useful prop in Rachel's case was the sight of a Scrabble board. Her Primary Theme was country dancing, but she also loved Scrabble and had often enjoyed playing it on her own in the past if she was short of a partner at the time. Again, Penny suggested that a Scrabble board be left out in the room and asked the carer what favourite word he might set out on the board to draw Rachel's interest in while he was away. After much discussion they settled on 'gavotte'. Penny explained that he needed an explanation for his own departure from the room that would leave Rachel on green and increase the chance that while he was away she would gravitate back to the familiarity of a gavotte via the Scrabble board.

You may think this is all a bit over-fussy but the dementia disability is nearly always far greater than the client lets on. They are truly at a loss, desperately seeking information. That is why they tend to wander around a lot, always searching: it is because they wonder. They wonder where you are, why you are absent, when you will be back: all sorts of things. It's because they're wondering that they start to wander, to try and find out. After all, they haven't lost their mobility or energy. They may be moving small things about, rearranging the trinkets on the mantelpiece, moving the crockery about in the kitchen, reorganising their clothes. There are two reasons why they may be doing this. They may be pottering about in a contemplative work mode, rather similar to Francis's wife at the jigsaw. They may, on the other hand, be attempting to find something they can sort out, and behind this realigning of the physical world may lie huge anxiety. If compulsively reorganising in a restless way, they are likely to be grappling with 'Where's my husband?', 'What is happening next?', 'What is the matter with me?' No sequences from today are complete, they have only fragments, hardly anything is intact. This is scary territory and may have been inhabited for minutes, hours, days or even months without any satisfactory resolution. They have been left wondering at some point and are more than likely to have been supplied with excessive, unmanageable factual detail by the carer before they left. Those facts don't store properly and for the umpteenth time the client is on amber heading for the disaster of a red blank. That is why Penny states that her aim for clients is that 'There must be nothing new under the sun. Life must go on for them in a way that they totally recognise. This means keeping everything in the present synchronised with the past.'

Regarding comings and goings, three kinds of repeatable and acceptable Explanations are essential if that is to be the case:

- The reason for the carer to be departing from the room.
- The reason that, once out of the room, the carer is absent – the explanation that will be provided to the client once the main carer has left the house.
- The reason why a substitute carer is there – the answer to the client's question 'Why doesn't this person who is with me go away and leave me alone? I really don't need them in the house.'

DEPARTURE EXPLANATION

Get out your notebook and write down as many Explanations as you can for why you might leave the room for a brief period, like five minutes. It's the kind of reason you would give if you prefaced it by saying 'I've got to slip off for a couple of minutes. Won't be long.'

Most Explanations that carers come up with are concerned with personal care of some sort, including 'going to the loo' or a similar toileting phrase. There have been many others developed by carers at Burford over the years including popping upstairs for a book, cooking a meal, putting the dog out, changing one's shirt, emptying the dishwasher. One to be avoided on your list is 'making a phone call'. Either answering or making a call contains much peril for the client as it raises a series of potentially disastrous questions in the client's mind, by which time the carer is out of the room and cannot provide reassuring answers to the client's inevitable questions – 'Who is calling?', 'What do they want?', and so on. Where there is a main carer living with the client, Penny advocates trying to keep phones and clients completely apart from each other.

You select the best explanation by the usual process of testing them out to see which seems most acceptable to the client: SPOTting. In choosing it, the key is that the client feels they are in control, that they are giving consent. The explanation offered should spark the following thoughts in the client's mind: 'Go on then, get on with it. You don't need me to do that. I'll be fine staying here.' You need to leave them feeling they have no further questions about this departure. The explanation is usually of a kind that would seem largely unnecessary in normal life. Suppose you were sitting with a friend watching TV. You might well not tell them you were going to the loo and if you did they would probably think 'That's more information than I need, just get on with it. Honestly, I don't need to know that. Feel free, carry on.' That is exactly the reaction you are looking for. You must have the feeling that they are dismissing you, sending you away to do whatever it is that you have to do and with no wish to join you. You leave behind you a sense of their being in control, that all is well with the world, even if they have little or no recollection of what you have said.

To test out which of your three Explanations is the best, try them out on successive days, giving a score out of 10 as to how much it passes the 'fine, get on with it' test.

Having settled on the best one, you need to start using this explanation over and over. The simpler it is, the better, and it needs some sort of characteristic gesture. As you introduce the words and gesture on a regular, repeating basis, you will find that the ritual becomes a customary part of the daily routine. In due course the words will become almost unnecessary – just the look, the wave, the pointed finger should become sufficient to leave the client feeling completely confident of what is going on. Once the explanation is established, the client is extremely unlikely to follow you because they have a powerful sense of being the one who has dismissed you, the one who wants you to leave, while, importantly, feeling that you are still very close at hand.

For example, Paul has identified that the best reason for his departure from Jan's presence is 'I need to smarten up.' Jan offers the marvellous response 'Good idea! Off you go! You look a right mess!' All the necessary elements we seek are present in Jan's statement. She is in control, sorting Paul out, sending him off, giving him consent to go. What a contrast to the carer who gets up to leave the room, either saying nothing or offering a battery of factual information which is completely lost on the client. Imagine if Paul said, 'I am going to make a telephone call to a chap who I am hoping is going to come and mend the drainpipe which is flooding the upstairs bathroom every time it rains. It's becoming a real problem.' That was the sort of factual information that Paul was liable to give to Jan before he developed SPECALSENSE. Jan would perhaps store less than half (often considerably less) of Paul's statement, and might end up with 'I am going . . . a real problem.' It might equally well end up as 'I am going to . . . who . . . going to come . . . which is every time . . .' Jan would be lumbered with a baffling array of new information that, if she did consult her album after he had left the room, would be at best muddling and at worst plain alarming. Small wonder that within moments of Paul having left the room to make his telephone call Jan would be coming to find him and interrupt with anxious questions.

Another example entailed a very useful prop. Carer Jocelyn only had to pick up his newspaper for it to indicate to his wife where he was going. This was already stored as an old photograph. He told

Penny that 'I don't like sitting on the loo without something to read because it always seems like a waste of time. She's used to this pattern from me that tells her that I'm not going far or will be a long time. She'll say "you're off to the loo" as soon as she sees me stand up and pick up the paper.' Penny pointed out that he should not underestimate how long she will stay on green once she has seen that acceptable explanation. Green endures once established. The more you can develop an explanation that is grounded in old green photographs, the less likely you are to trigger insecurity and the longer the positive feelings will remain accessible after the explanation for your departure. For example, James was a retired banker, and hated wasting money. His wife had only to tell him she was going to check there were no lights left on in the house and he was as happy as Larry. The feeling of being in control of his money buoyed him up in an enduring way, although the facts she had given him had not stored at all.

ABSENCE EXPLANATION

The Absence Explanation is necessary so that a substitute carer can reassure the client about where the main carer has gone. It's important to note that the explanation for the carer's departure and the one for their absence – supplied by a substitute carer – are not the same thing. The departure one is supplied by you as main carer, and is all about being of minimal interest and triggering 'just get on with it!'; the absence one works because the client feels relieved that you are engaged in something either 'useful' or that you enjoy, and is supplied by whoever is there instead. The two Explanations need to be different because one implies that you will be returning soon from within the house, and is given by you; whereas the other carries the message that you are away from the house for some time, and is provided by someone else.

This time write down some places where you might have gone away from home in the past for several hours, or even a day – the office, the golf course, the hairdresser, and so on. Now pick the most reassuring explanation for why you would be there. This time, you are looking for one that makes the client feel 'Phew, thank goodness I haven't had to go too!' and 'Great, that will be good for him and will have desirable consequences.' It needs to be something the client thinks the carer will want to do and something that the client is happy not to get involved in. It also needs to be off the premises.

For instance, one carer wrote down various options: 'going to the DIY store', 'going to the travel agent' and 'going to my shed at the end of the garden'. Penny advised against the travel agent because it ran the risk of being something the client might like to do too. They took all their holidays together and the client used to make all the decisions. The shed was no good because it was within a minute's walking distance from the house, and the client might well want to go and look if they were told that the carer was there. The DIY shopping trip was best because it was something of no direct interest to the client but which would indirectly please them. The carer used verbal ping-pong to find the best item of shopping required and discovered that 'bathroom tiles' scored best. Apparently there was a cracked tile in the bathroom which the client kept pointing out. By using tiles as the Explanation for Absence, the client responded, time after time, with 'At least he's doing something useful at last!' Penny advocated that the carer didn't rush to mend the tile, as a broken one was a marvellous prop to reinforce this explanation.

Another simple instance was 'pottery', used by Joy for her

husband Tom. She used to make enormous pots that Tom greatly admired – this had been so for the past 30 years. The kiln was not in their (small) cottage and she had always had to go out in order to do pottery, so he was quite happy with the explanation.

A more unusual example was a carer wife whose husband did not relish the explanation that the destination was for her own enjoyment, like the theatre. He had always rather disapproved of the entertainment world and he found it much more acceptable to know that she was doing something 'useful'. Possibilities included looking after the grandchildren and helping with the local church, but the best of all was shopping for food. So long as she remembered the wine, that was fine by him.

Mathew was a similar illustration of a self-interested husband. 'Nursing stuff' was the Absence Explanation used by his wife Sylvia. One of Mathew's favourite sayings was 'I married a nurse', as that showed great foresight for being looked after by her in the future, so he was delighted to think she was off brushing up her nursing skills in some way which would ultimately benefit him. This was like an insurance policy for him, as a former banker and admirer of shrewd fiscal planning. In this particular case, Sylvia used a variant of the nursing context for her Explanation for Departure, 'washing hands', that old-fashioned and much-needed activity for nurses of which Mathew again thoroughly approved. Interestingly, some time after Mathew had moved to a nursing home, Sylvia herself became a client; her son, by now the main carer, selected 'Nursing in the *old* way' as his mother's Primary Theme. This was accompanied by the phrase 'Things ain't what they used to be', and a gesture of holding the thumb and index finger in a circle and making as if to throw a dart, to denote an old-fashioned way of giving a painless injection using an orange for practice.

At its best, the Explanation for Absence actually boosts the client's well-being. Peter would feel relaxed if he knew that his carer wife Mavis was 'out with the girls', a familiar activity that Peter would not wish to deprive her of and which could not possibly for a moment involve him. But Mavis's surefire absence winner turned out to be 'doing something with my parents', which carried the message that she was in the Midlands and out of reach; at the same time she was defined as gainfully employed taking care of her elderly and frail parents. Peter knew from many years back that unless Mavis kept in close touch with her parents, she would be anxious and unhappy. Played carefully, this 'parents' plan also boosted Peter's well-being because it conveyed that he was not the one needing looking after and that he was being unselfish in settling for her doing things for others rather than being with him. However, in talking things through with Mavis, Penny encountered a not uncommon problem.

Mavis was prone to conflating the Explanation for Departure with the one for absence. It was only after a considerable number of botches that she realised the importance of the substitute carer only using the 'parents' explanation when Mavis needed to be away for some time. Mavis's Departure Explanation, required only for brief partings, was 'checking up on the food in the kitchen'. If she used the explanation of going to the Midlands as she walked out of the door, Peter would become caught up in all the details of how long she was going to be away and when she was coming back again, and become very anxious indeed. It was crucial to use the 'checking up on the food in the kitchen' for leaving, allowing the substitute carer to provide information about the Midlands after she had left the house.

While it is not essential, it is helpful if an Absence Explanation derives from the client's Primary Theme. It is sometimes possible to carve something out. For example, Betty's absence was best explained by her daughter being out at the other end of their small-holding checking the chickens. Betty's Primary Theme was 'making ends meet' at which she had excelled, particularly during the war. The chickens represented her livelihood, her means of keeping the family fed, having lost her husband during the war. She had a bad hip dating from a long time back and this provided the Health Theme. Being told that her daughter was 'seeing to the chickens' usually triggered Betty to say that she didn't know what she would do without her daughter, given her own dodgy hip. There was no way Betty was ever going to want to stagger down the fields to join her daughter. Eventually, Penny introduced neighbours and friends who called in to ask Betty's advice about something to do with chickens – either they were thinking of keeping chickens them-selves, or they were complaining about how dreadful the shop eggs had become. Penny managed to get chickens introduced everywhere in Betty's life in the end, although the daughter was fairly sceptical to start with. Of course, a Red-to-Green Loop was needed in case Betty landed on the old red of her husband's death while travelling along the chickens-and-the-war conversational pathway. This loop was easy to develop because there was so much she admired about her husband whose life had been cut short before the honeymoon period of her marriage was over. Betty could soon be brought back from the sadness of loss to gladness about what she had known, in a way which would have been far more difficult if she had not been a client.

EXPLANATION FOR THE PRESENCE OF A SUBSTITUTE CARER

The Explanation for Departure is a subject of no interest to the client ('Just go ahead') and that for absence is something that seems a pleasing use of the carer's time ('Jolly good, glad they're getting on with it'). The explanation you now need involves a problem that the substitute carer can mention to the client in the hope that the client can help out. That way the substitute won't be shown the door. The Explanation for Presence always links to the Primary Theme, at least to start with. The problem which the substitute carer would like help with needs to be one which comes from old photographs, known to be accessed regularly through ping-pong and triggered by a particular catchphrase or a physical prop or gesture.

What we are looking for is something connected with the Primary Theme which the client feels only they understand or have the answers to. With the main carer absent, when the client says, 'Who are you?' or 'What are you doing here?' to the substitute, the answer needs to be something which makes perfect sense and conveys the feeling that this person has popped in to get their advice in an area where they feel less than completely at home.

To find the most useful problem for the substitute carer to offer, you SPOT in the usual way, jotting down three problems that might work and then testing each one out for a day, scoring it from 1 to 10, to see how much it satisfies the client. To get a feel for the right sort of thing, try a few sentences beginning 'I feel a bit stupid that I don't know whether . . .' and then add a point of fact that you know the client knows about and is still accessing from old photos. Whether it's fire engines or rugby or raising chickens, it should not be hard to establish a basic issue a substitute carer could mention as their problem and which would set the client off happily explaining. It needs to be something that is sufficiently popular with the client that it can be repeated again and again – that should be an important criterion when scoring its suitability. If the client appears bored it's a sure sign it is not the right one. You want something that a complete stranger can raise with the client and which can be almost guaranteed to provoke a stream of commentary.

For example, Robert delighted in explaining the difference between a swallow and a swift to pretty well anyone, provided they sounded authentically interested, bird watching being his Primary Theme. Penny settled on the swallow and the swift because of the length and richness of Robert's response each time, and the ease with which they could move on to other things, with Penny knowing that she could re-launch it quite simply if she needed to, via a well-worn conversational pathway. It needs to be a cracker because the carer is going to have to get other people to use it during their absence – bull's-eye stuff, a known winner.

For instance, Grace was happy to advise between a choice of two different styles of handbag – decorative versus functional. Years before his death, her husband had made bags. Grace was devoted to his memory and always carried one particular bag around with her as she was just so proud of it, telling you in minute detail how each bit had been lovingly made. If anyone was sitting with Grace while her daughter was away, saying something about not being sure of one's handbag – wondering whether it was any good or should perhaps be replaced – was known to trigger Grace's story. Showing her a particular picture of the two types of bag in a women's magazine was the most reliable prompt of all. The phrase each visitor used was 'I'm having a bit of a handbag problem' and Grace was immediately engaged. Before the explanation was developed there had been many problems whenever anyone came to sit with her. But once it had been developed, she never queried that person's presence while her daughter was away. Often the best opening shot was to say that the catch was not working properly (Grace would tell you that her own handbag catch was of the finest, chosen specially by her dear late husband). Get her on the subject of her husband via your handbag and she was away all over again. All the best people carried handbags in Grace's view, so it became an easy problem for all her visitors to discuss, whether women or men.

On top of the Departure, Absence and Presence Explanations, there is one final tool you need for smooth management of all situations. It is required in case of emergency and a vital back-up in case the Health Theme should fail. Its purpose is to rein in the client from damaging behaviour or states of mind when everything else has been tried.

THE ALTRUISTIC TRIGGER

There will always be a risk that the client decides to get up and go somewhere on their own, or to do something else which could be dangerous, like getting into the driving seat of a car with keys in its ignition. Despite being unsafe and inconvenient to other people, the client is determined to go ahead. Explanations based on the Primary and Health Themes have failed: this is a major crisis. The client is saying, 'I am leaving, get out my way: no one is going to stop me.' Physical restraint would distress the client in a potentially catastrophic way, ramming home to them the extent of their disempowerment and disability, to the point of abuse. With the utmost urgency, you need a bottom-line strategy. Penny calls it the Altruistic Trigger.

As with everything else, Penny first discovered its necessity through Dorothy. Dorothy and Sam had been staying with Penny for Christmas. It had been a difficult few days, as Dorothy was becoming increasingly distressed in Sam's company, particularly when she was alone with him. His use of common sense was doing the harm, trying to keep her up to the (his) mark.

They were due to go on to stay with a friend before returning to their home. Penny tried desperately to persuade Dorothy to stay on with her while Sam went to see their friend on his own. Sam insisted on asking Dorothy's view of this arrangement himself. As soon as he asked, 'Would you really prefer to stay here while I go to Shropshire on my own?' Dorothy was completely thrown. Penny could see that she wasn't sure what 'Shropshire' would entail and that she was not clear whether her answer should be yes or no. The powerful pull of duty towards Sam won out and there was nothing Penny could do. Dorothy went off looking hugely strained, and the visit was seriously unsuccessful. When Penny next saw her, some weeks later, there had been an observable downward step in her overall ability to cope with life: she was battered, emotionally and physically, by what had occurred. The experience taught Penny that extreme damage can result from being unable to negotiate with the client to achieve a safe option on their behalf.

It took much pondering before Penny discovered how to introduce an explanation to the client as to why they should ignore their natural inclination to do something and to accept another course of action. This Altruistic Trigger was needed again and again as Penny worked to persuade clients not to leave Burford Hospital when they were staying overnight and it was also crucial for the care home when the client first moved there from the family home. Repeatedly, wherever they were, she would be faced with a despairing or confused client who had decided they had had enough and were going home now. What was needed was a way of making an offer to the client that they could not refuse.

Altruism emerged over the years as the answer: when the client is able to realise that if they pursue their chosen course it will cause great problems for someone they care about, they give way and feel good about doing so.

For example, Rita was a particularly troublesome client whose Primary Theme was actually grumbling – give her one of her favourite gripes to talk about and she was away. However, she was extremely fond of her daughter, who was a single parent and made soft furnishings for a living. Rita greatly admired her daughter's capacity to fend for herself and it turned out that she would do almost anything to avoid causing loss of income or angst to her daughter. Hence, if Rita reached the crisis point during an overnight stay at the hospital and declared she was leaving right there and then, it was only necessary to tell her that her daughter would be so worried that she would feel obliged to leave an important job she had on at that moment. The catchphrase was 'hanging curtains', which Rita knew from old as being a time-consuming and difficult job. She had no wish whatsoever to upset her daughter or cause her to lose money and this was sufficiently powerful to persuade her to change her mind.

Penny worked out an Altruistic Trigger for Dorothy which was helpful when she moved into the nursing home. Sam had suffered for many years from a cortisone deficiency – Addison's disease – and could become very exhausted and depressed. As soon as Dorothy knew that she was being asked to do something in order that 'Sam's Addison's disease doesn't get any worse' she was more than happy to fall in with whatever suggestion was being made.

Some readers may feel this strategem crosses the line between helpful guidance and deceit: misleading a cognitively impaired, powerless person who must depend on the honesty of others. In the case of Rita, did her carer deliberately trick her into believing that her daughter would suffer a financial penalty if Rita pursued her chosen path?

When they have such thoughts, readers must remind themselves of Penny's advice regarding client consent: grow up and be robust. The only question you should ask is 'What would you have a carer do if you were a client? What would the client want you to do if they had all their faculties and could be presented with the conundrum?' Clearly, the answer is that the Altruistic Trigger is completely for the client's good, that it is a choice between the client being perfectly contented with the world or in a state of potentially catastrophic distress. That is, as they say, a no-brainer if you have the client's best interests at heart. The Altruistic Trigger is rarely used but is an essential part of 24-hour wraparound care.

TROUBLESHOOTING

'My father has lived on his own for many years, and I always say goodbye when it is time to leave. He seems quite happy to wave me off. Surely the Explanation for Departure should indicate to him that I am leaving rather than staying on somewhere in the house?'
There are some key differences between people who live on their own (particularly if they have done so for a long time) and those who share their home with another person. Some people who live on their own are known to enjoy the peace and quiet of their home once their visitors have departed, particularly if they are not constantly plagued by anxious questions once they are alone. SPOT will tell you whether

your father is waving you off out of politeness, or whether he is genuinely content and confident about the future as you depart. In this situation you need to identify a phrase which covers both departure and absence, carrying with it the message that you are close at hand whenever he needs you. The key factor here is to reduce the information about distance and time to a minimum, so that you retain the best elements of 'I'm just popping off for a while and everything will be fine while I am temporarily out of sight.' The phrase you use on a repeating basis will serve you well if and when your father ever moves into a formal care setting. The feeling that you are close at hand will always be with him, wherever he is at the time.

'Surely I don't have to offer the Explanation for Departure to my husband every single time I leave the room?'
Once you have found the Explanation for Departure, you need to be thinking about it yourself every time you leave the room. Consider what cues you are giving about where you are going, even if you don't say anything at all. For instance, if SPOT has highlighted that your husband is delighted to think that you are off to the kitchen, start thinking of the gesture that might convey that idea. Perhaps an apron would be handy, either worn or lying on a chair ready to be picked up. Perhaps a recipe book would be a useful prop to pick up as you leave. Perhaps the gesture of dusting your hand against your skirt, as if it were an apron, will convey a useful message in a remarkably economic way. Also, you can focus each time you leave on the art of evaporating – almost melting away – leaving only a feeling of security behind. It is the repetition and recycling of feelings, in yourself as much as in your husband, which is so valuable and will pay so many dividends in the future.

'I have mentioned the Explanation for Presence to my neighbour who sometimes pops in, and she now seems really worried about what she is going to say and do when she comes.'

It is important to consider the 'need to know', and your neighbour only really needs to be given a tip as to a good line of conversation that you have uncovered, and that all visitors are now aiming to use. Provided the neighbour understands the value of repetition, and learns to love it herself, she will become more confident, not less, each time she pops in. You need to relay really simple information to other members of your team. The information will be based on all your work to develop the Profile (see Chapter 10), but there's no need to baffle everyone else with the science of it all. Keep it as simple as possible!

'The whole idea of using the Altruistic Trigger worries me so much that I am finding it difficult to start finding out what it might be. What should I do?'

There is an important positive aspect to the Altruistic Trigger in that we would all rather help someone else with a problem they have than feel we have a problem ourselves. The Altruistic Trigger offers a way forward for the client when they are feeling most up against it, and it really can offer a feeling of satisfaction to them at an otherwise challenging moment. Like all other aspects of the Profile (see Chapter 10), the Altruistic Trigger has been shown over the years to be essential if and when the client moves into formal care, and you will not be able to identify and develop it overnight. Forward planning is everything here, and your carer courage must come to the fore!

TO IDENTIFY ACCEPTABLE EXPLANATIONS FOR
DEPARTURE, ABSENCE AND PRESENCE

DEPARTURE

1. Think of the many reasons why you might have to leave the room for a few moments.

2. Try out each one on the client and SPOT which one causes the client to dismiss you with confidence, rather than appearing concerned.

3. When you have found the best answer, use it all the time.

ABSENCE

1. Think about the many reasons why you have been away from the house in the past.

2. Talk casually with the client about a possible plan you have for doing each of the activities on your list. Use SPOT to evaluate which topics generate the most enthusiasm from the client. Score most points for the one which causes the client to say, 'Oh Good! I'm glad about that! How lovely!'

3. Write that one down and ensure that anyone with the client uses it to explain your absence whenever the client asks where you are.

PRESENCE OF A THIRD PARTY IN YOUR ABSENCE

1. Ask anyone who spends time with the client to SPOT how many times the question of your absence is asked.

2. Bring into your mind your client's Primary Theme, and add the crucial prop to your mental picture.

3. Consider what sort of problem your substitute carer might have which the client might like to help with.

4. Try out various endings to the following sentence: 'I feel a bit

stupid but I really don't quite understand about . . .' with your client and SPOT the results.

5. Decide on the best one and ask anyone who is with the client to use that technique to provide a context for their presence.

6. Ask the person to show over-the-top gratitude and admiration for the client.

CHAPTER TEN

The Care Profile

This chapter pulls together the various skills you have learned up to now in Part Two. Let's start by recapitulating the essentials for providing 24-hour wraparound care.

THE ESSENTIALS

Penny Garner divides feelings into green (the normal experience until dementia appears on the scene) and unacceptable red (deep trauma which is extremely rare indeed in normal life). In the absence of dementia we are well placed to deal with a red when it enters our life: we have the facts and can take action. This ability to cope with red changes dramatically and potentially disastrously when dementia enters the scene.

To protect from new red is the SPECAL carer's primary goal. This goal is what provides the carer with consent to support the client's version of reality and to buttress it as necessary. There are three fundamental commandments for doing so: Thou Shalt Not Ask Questions (play ping-pong instead); Thou Shalt Learn From The

Client (using SPOT to identify the most productive answers to repeated questions); and Thou Shalt Always Agree With The Client (via the Red-to-Green Conversational Loop).

What converts these commandments into wraparound care is the Primary Theme. Since clients still have full access to many old photographs, identifying the most satisfactory set of photographs as the foundation of their daily experience is vital. Catchphrases, physical props and gestures will increasingly be all that is required to trigger the theme as the illness progresses.

However, it is also vital to have a Health Theme to orientate the client when everyday, present realities have to be navigated, such as making a transition from one place (e.g., the sitting room or the lavatory) or activity (e.g., watching telly or going to bed) to another.

A single explanation in each case is also required for the departure and the absence of the carer, and for the presence of any substitute carers.

In the event of an emergency situation, one in which the client is determined upon a course of action which could be dangerous or unacceptable, an Altruistic Trigger needs to have been identified.

CREATING A CLIENT CARE PROFILE OUT OF THE ESSENTIALS

With these points in mind, it is time to set down on paper the particulars of your client's Care Profile. You need this to remind yourself of the basic techniques you now have at your disposal. Write down each of the following for your client:

Primary Theme: Its title or catchphrase, a collection of significant cue words and a brief summary – only a couple of lines – of what it is about. Any physical props or gestures which connote it.

Health Theme: Its title or catchphrase, the key words which summarise the background story and the physical props or gestures which connote it.

Departure Explanation: Its title or catchphrase, physical props and gestures.

Absence Explanation: Its title or catchphrase, physical props and gestures.

Presence Explanation: Its title or catchphrase, physical props and gestures.

Altruistic Trigger: Its title or catchphrase, follow-on information, and gesture.

Most frequently asked client questions and SPOTted answers

Before you go any further have a look at the following background information about a SPECAL client called Fred.

Profile for Fred
Fred is a keen rugby player who used to play for his village team and is an avid supporter of Wasps as well as England. He refers to a coffee

break as 'half time'. He also used to play cricket and was hit in the knee by a cricket ball in his youth. He had intensive physiotherapy which sorted the knee out, but he has always had to be careful not to overdo things. He always assumes anyone leaving the room carrying a book or a newspaper is heading for the bathroom. His wife Joan is a keen golfer. She took up golf years ago on the advice of her heart surgeon and Fred is keen that she takes care of her health. Joan tends to worry about Fred and although her fussing annoys Fred hugely, he will do anything rather than upset her.

Primary Theme: 'Rugby' – Fred was a keen rugby player.

Key words: Weston, Wasps, rugger buggers, Harlequins, fly half, Hereford, England, props, scrum, maul, posts, 25, try, match, 15, side, end, stands, tackling, dressing room, shirts, referee, tickets, six nations, half time, full time, blow the whistle, linesmen, Wales, national anthem, singing, haka . . .

Props: Pillow shaped like a rugger ball. Yellow and black striped coffee mug.

Gesture: Smooth sideways swoop of the arms, hands holding imaginary ball and then letting it go.

Health Theme: Dodgy knee.

Key words: 'Diogenes disease!', 'the get-fit quack', 'best not stir up the old bones'.

Gesture: Flexing of leg to demonstrate restricted movement.

Departure Explanation: 'Just going to the loo.'

Props: Folded newspaper or book, either carried or left on chair.

Gesture: Fold the newspaper or check book marker while rising from chair, sideways nod of the head with eye-contact.

Absence Explanation: 'Gone to golf.'

Prop: Golf club left in the hall – 'She's gone to get a new one.'

Gesture: Feet apart, arms held together out in front, to swing imaginary club.

Presence Explanation: Problem choosing between Wasps and Harlequins as the better club.

Prop: Newspaper with a sports page featuring rugby.

Altruistic Trigger: 'Joan will be *so* worried.'

Gesture: Hand across chest suggesting *mea culpa.*

Most frequently asked client questions and SPOTted answers:

1. Where's Joan? – Gone to play golf
2. Where's my car? – Being overhauled
3. What's for supper? – Something hot

The main point of writing this Profile down is to fix it in your mind so that you can begin using it each day, a useful aide-memoire for when you are feeling tired or rattled. It will inspire you to keep an ongoing record of vocabulary and quotes as you develop a small dictionary of special words. To start with you will be using words that you already know from long ago to have connotations for the client. As you go on developing your basic database of favourite words and phrases, you will start to spot connections between the words and routine activities of daily life. You can begin to try them out and use them to play verbal ping-pong. Because you now understand the ideas that lie behind each element, you will soon find you are automatically putting the Profile to use, almost without thinking. Bear in mind that the client is still (and always will be) storing some new full photographs (not just feelings but facts as well). Although the trend over the years will be towards less and less storage, even in the latest stages some storage does still occur. If you are constantly using the same tried and tested words and phrases, these will store at least at the level of feelings, even if not as facts. This ensures new green.

Interestingly, when the Royal College of Nursing carried out an evaluation of SPECAL, they found that carers were reporting that the memory loss of the client appeared to plateau. This was due to the repetition of old material that was storing so much more effectively than new. There is a huge amount conjured up for Fred in the words 'half time', all the joys of rugby and what that has meant to him. These two words, repeated in context at mealtimes, will occasionally be stored, and will mean so much more to Fred than a statement of 'Come along, Fred, we must go downstairs for breakfast. It's Tuesday and the gas man may be calling to repair the cooker.' Fred will not store even half of that new data, whereas if 'half time' is recycled in the right tone of voice every time a meal or snack is in the immediate offing, it has a far higher chance of storage. Even if it doesn't store, it will do the trick.

The Care Profile can also be used to help when coaching helpers. As the person who has devised the Profile, you are the principal person upon whom the client's well-being hinges. Simple bits of information can be extracted from the Profile as you coach people who will come into contact with the client or who may also act as carer in your place. What remains is to explain how you employ this Profile in enabling everyone who comes into contact with the client to help them or, at the least, not to upset them. This is the subject of the next chapter and of Part Three.

CHAPTER ELEVEN

Identify and Manage your Team

In some respects this is the most important chapter in the whole book because it explains how to avoid becoming hopelessly isolated as a main carer. If you go it alone and expect to provide 24-hour wraparound care single-handedly for the rest of the client's life, you will go bonkers or suffer a physical collapse. Penny Garner introduced the term 'carer's dementia' when she first started working at Burford, to describe the desperate state most carers were in by the time the client was referred. It is absolutely essential for both client and carer well-being to create a team, with you as the manager. This chapter explains how to pick that team and train it.

PRIMING *EVERYONE* IN THE CLIENT'S SOCIAL WORLD TO AVOID RED

It may not have occurred to you until now but if you stop to think about it, anyone who is not aware of the basics of SPECALCARE has the potential to create a catastrophic red for the client. Visitors who spend time in the client's company are inevitably operating according to common sense, not SPECALSENSE. If the next door neighbour or your visiting cousin has not had any preparation, they are bound to ask questions, like 'How are you feeling?' or 'Have you been playing any Bridge?' When the client responds with statements that are 'wrong', such as 'Tony Blair is the Prime Minister' or that their (long dead) dog Raffles is out playing in the garden, the visitor is very liable to disagree. If the client asks the same question five times or repeatedly tells the same story, although the visitor may have the diplomacy to not openly draw attention to the repetitiveness, without special instruction they are almost bound to show by their body language that something is very wrong and that they are becoming bored as well as embarrassed. All of these scenarios could be disastrous. The only way to be sure of avoiding them is to anticipate every single person the client is going to come into contact with and give them a two-minute crash course in SPECAL basics. On no account should you leave the client alone with someone who has no such training, within seconds things could go horribly wrong.

This is not to counsel total social isolation; in fact, the opposite is advocated. You should try and ensure that anyone who would have come into pleasurable social contact with the client in the days before dementia struck, is still able to do so. It is simply to stress the importance of regulation of the client's social environs. The more people in your circle who understand the rock-bottom basics of what is required for wraparound care, the safer, and the more rewarding for those who visit.

In most cases, when dementia is diagnosed there is an initial flurry of friends and relatives feeling that they ought to find some way to help. Their reactions are often informed by the negativity of the press coverage. At best they will be sympathetic; at worst, terrified and depressed. Many err on the side of avoiding contact, if they possibly can. However, there will be visits as well as phone calls from intimates and the closer friends to see how the client and carer are getting on. While it is really important to sustain the social infra-structure of the client's life and your own, visits made without any preparation will leave the client feeling threatened and exposed. At the same time the visitors are liable to become scared, feel embarrassed and mournful that their much-loved old friend or relative is obviously never going to recover. Whether consciously or not, the visitor is liable to feel that the client they knew has died and fail to see what they can do to make a difference. There follows a rapid and depressing reduction in the social circle, with many looser acquaintances losing touch altogether and the phone calls from intimates becoming fewer and fewer. As the circle constricts, the carer feels increasingly strangled. The next Christmas card sent out by the carer is likely to contain deeply melancholic sentiments along the lines of 'Sadly George has this awful illness and prospects are not great, but we are doing our best in the circumstances.' No one receiving that card is going to feel particularly uplifted at the prospect of their next visit, and indeed hardly knows what to write back in reply.

Yet it need not be that way with SPECALSENSE and the right preparation. SPECAL carers are encouraged to spread the news that although the client has a memory disability, nothing has really changed because the carer has found a new and remarkably effective method of managing the condition in ways which keep everyone reasonably content. A typical quote from a SPECAL carer is 'My wife's dementia is far worse but it really doesn't seem to matter very much. We're all fine.'

IDENTIFYING THE PLAYERS

To get to this point, you will need to consider all the potential players in your team. We are using the word 'team' here in the broadest possible sense, to include everyone who comes into contact with the client. Ultimately, there are going to be two different categories. There are the people who have only casual or occasional contact, who need only basic preparation. They are very unlikely indeed to spend time with the client on their own. Then there is the core care delivery team, the people who spend some time with the client when you, as main carer, are elsewhere. This group needs more advanced preparation.

Apart from how much time they spend with the client, the simplest way to distinguish core and occasional categories is to decide whether or not they will ever be left alone with the client. With remarkably little training, the core members will be able to substitute for you because they will understand the basics of the Primary Theme. I will come to the syllabi of the basic and advanced kinds of preparation presently, but before that, to establish who is who, you need three pages in your notebook.

On the first, put 'relatives' at the top and write down every member of your own and the client's family that either of you have ever met. Beside each name put a mark which indicates those that you see less than once a year, those more than once a year and ones who you believe would want to be part of decision-making processes involving the client's care. The third category of decision-makers is an important one when it comes to choosing a nursing home, and we will look at that in detail in Part Three. The first two categories will probably require basic preparation; the third will require the advanced kind. Place a B for basic or an A for advanced preparation beside each name, as appropriate.

Now put 'friends, neighbours, acquaintances and tradespeople' at the top of the next page and list every single one you can think of. Now put a B or an A (basic or advanced preparation) beside each name, as necessary, the simplest criterion being whether the client is ever going to be left alone with them.

Finally, write 'professionals' at the top of your third page. These are likely to include any or all of the following: GP, consultant, community psychiatric nurse, community nurse, clinical psychologist, physiotherapist, occupational therapist, speech and language therapist, care manager/social services contact, carers' support services, paid home help, nursing or other agency services, nursing home manager or assistant, Alzheimer's Society, Age Concern or other non-governmental organisation support. Using the criterion of whether you are ever going to leave the client alone with this professional, put A or B beside each name.

This exercise often surprises people. Carers feel that they are on their own, that there are few others around to help. Yet all the names on your various lists represent people who are *already* coming into contact with the client, however rarely.

Having done this exercise, you are ready to prepare both categories to play for your team.

BASIC PREPARATION FOR THE 'B' GROUP

This is done by a short chat using a few well-chosen words, sometimes combined with written information (see page 206). The goal is to convey the rudiments of the three commandments: don't ask questions, learn from the expert, always agree.

Overleaf is a summary sheet of 'Important Information' of what the 'B' group needs to know. Preferably, create an opportunity to discuss this summary with them before they next meet the client, in case they have any queries. Ideally you would send it to them before the encounter, although that is not always possible and you should always have a spare copy available on your person in case they have not received it or not read it. You can download the summary from the SPECAL website (www.specal.co.uk), or if you do not have access to the Internet or do not have a printer, you can photocopy it. Failing that, SPECAL can send you some copies if you contact them at: The SPECAL Centre, Sheep Street, Burford OX18 4SL.

Important Information

You are about to meet . . . . and there are a few things I would ask you to take into account when talking with them.

This person has a disability which makes it hard or impossible to store new factual information, although they experience and store feelings in the normal way. Apart from this, they are exactly the same person as they used to be but their disability does require a few basic adjustments to how you communicate with them.

1. Please do not ask them any direct questions at all. If you require factual information, please obtain it from me as their advocate. If you are paying a social call, please abstain from quizzing them about anything whatsoever – any such queries have the potential to be extremely confusing or distressing. Instead, please bear in mind that . . . . is particularly interested in . . . . and is most likely to engage with you if you use the following phrases set out below:

Subject   Phrases

2. If . . . . repeats themselves, such as asking the same question several times or telling a story more than once, please take care not to point this out to them either by deed or word. From their standpoint, this is the first time they have said it and you will perturb them if you convey to them that you have heard it before. Instead, you may find that raising one of the subjects listed above, using the associated phrases, leads to a more productive exchange. Try to stop talking as soon as they start, and show your interest by body language rather than too many words.

3. If the client says something with which you disagree, please take care *not* to contradict them in word or deed. Because they have a particular memory problem and are having trouble storing new information, some of the things they say may seem wrong to you. But if you insist on your version of what is right you could be doing harm and you will certainly achieve no good.

4. . . . . may find it perplexing if you tell them about bad things that have happened to you or to others in the wider world. If you can convey cheerfulness and tell them that all is well with the world, that things are going well, things generally tend to go better for them.

Many thanks for your attention and I hope you enjoy getting together with . . . .!

Signature of main carer/advocate:

Before you engage in any preparations, it's worth checking that it is actually in the client's interest for the meeting to occur at all. Surprisingly often, the answer is 'no'. For example, there may be potentially problematic contacts with professionals that can be avoided. One carer told Penny she was dreading an appointment with a consultant because he was liable to ask so many red-threatening questions. Penny asked what the purpose of the session was and the carer said, 'Absolutely none, a pointless check-up.' Penny replied, 'So why are you going?' The carer said, 'It's been in the diary for ages, we've got no choice really', but Penny suggested she give the matter further thought. When the carer decided to call up the consultant's secretary and asked if it was all right to cancel, she was told they were delighted to get a free space and that the client's care would in no way be compromised by not attending. Another carer rang Penny to ask how best to get her client mother to Scotland to visit her other daughter, the carer's sister, even though she knew it could be disastrous. Again, Penny's question was why was the mother going, to which the reply was 'My sister likes having her. It suits her but I realise it's bad news for my mother.' Again, Penny counselled a review. After discussion the sister decided to come south to see her mother instead.

In an ideal world, the client would not have words addressed to them by anyone who has not had some kind of prior preparation. Obviously, some contacts with strangers are inevitable. You will sometimes find yourself in a supermarket or on a bus, and the checkout girl or a passenger will address a question to the client. It's up to you to quickly regain control of the situation by making the client feel part of the 'we' club alongside you. You and the client are the partnership, and the third party is just that, a third party outside rather than inside the relationship. At the supermarket, you might manoeuvre yourself subtly into position between the client and the checkout and say 'Please ask me the questions, and I will answer for us', including the client with a wave and a smile. In taking such assertive action, you might remind yourself of how thick-skinned you need to be when caring for small children and ignoring the crowd's censure as your toddler throws a tantrum.

While you can never guarantee what will happen with strangers or passers-by, there is a long list of other people that you can prepare. At its most basic, there is nothing to stop you catching the postman or milkman in the drive one morning and having a quiet word. They would far prefer to have an explanation of how they can help, rather than be left wondering what, if anything, they ought to be saying or doing. You might say the client 'is fine generally, but it's best if you do happen to come across them to restrict yourself to a smile and something positive. Try and keep all negative news out of the way – they tend to worry for days if they hear something depressing. Preferably don't regale them with "I was late for work this morning, there was this ghastly accident on the main road . . ."' The same advice can be delivered to some tradespeople. As much as possible, visit the same shops each time when out with your client, preferably small ones whose staff remain the same, like your local grocery store or post office, if you are lucky enough to have one. You can nip in and have a quiet word with likely looking serving staff.

Whether in this kind of exchange or engaged in meatier stuff, as a manager motivating a team you have to think continually of how to find ways to enable the player to be authentic and to be natural in dealing with the client. Be very careful not to give the team too much detail, as they quickly get swamped. If it's too programmatic, they get nervous and will not 'perform' well, and that is quickly picked up by the client who is ever sensitive to feelings and will become apprehensive themselves. It's a difficult balancing act, trying to flag up to people whom you may not know very well that common sense is not helpful and at the same time, keeping the player feeling confident rather than alarmed, unconfident or bamboozled.

Professionals form a large proportion of the people who are only occasionally in contact with the client. The most vital one is the GP and Penny recommends that the carer pay a separate visit without the client present, to seek their cooperation and understanding. It is essential that the GP sees the carer in an advocacy role with the consent of the client. Once the crucial issue of confidentiality has been satisfactorily resolved, the carer should hand the 'Important Information' sheet to the GP for immediate reading. The carer should explain that they will do their best to provide all factual information that the doctor may need. The carer will need to persuade them that they have the client's best interests at heart and show how helpful and time-saving they want to be. Most professionals are only too happy for help with cases of dementia, being all too often overstretched and eager for any assistance going.

If the doctor wishes to examine the client in person, the carer uses the Health Theme to ease the way. The doctor can be told beforehand what this is so that they can join in. They should understand how it makes for an easier life for the client to use it and is a better route for obtaining information that may be needed. The same formula should be followed with other professionals who will not be alone with the client. The community psychiatric nurse, the meals-on-wheels delivery person, all these kinds of categories can be given the 'Important Information' sheet and briefed out of the client's earshot. As with other team players, it's important to do it in a way that does not overload or worry them, so that they can be confident in dealing with the client. The client will readily pick up on their feelings and needs to know that they are relaxed.

The same preparation is required for friends or neighbours who are occasional visitors. However, with these it is worth keeping an eye out for any who might possibly be able at a later date to move to join the advanced players. Since you are hoping, if humanly or practically possible, never to leave the client alone unattended in the house, friends or neighbours may be able and willing to act as temporary carers if you need to nip out briefly to the hairdresser or to post a package.

ADVANCED PREPARATION FOR THE 'A' GROUP

This is required only for the core care team members: people you leave the client alone with, and are most likely to be relatives, close friends or paid helpers.

You need to convey to them that you have found a very helpful method for increasing the client's well-being: SPECAL. You would like them to learn it too and the best way is for them to read this book. You can lend them this copy or borrow it from the library. When they have finished, they will almost certainly have some useful suggestions regarding the Care Profile. You should give them the one you have prepared, as described in the last chapter, for discussion. In all probability, you and your team will find yourselves engaged in an absorbing discussion around the Primary and Health Themes chosen for your client, as well as the Explanations for Departure, Absence and Presence of Others, and the Altruistic Trigger that you have developed. Discussing these with other interested people can help to make SPECALCARE work for everyone in quite a short space of time.

THE CARER'S NEW PROJECT

Applied properly, the basic and advanced preparation of different team members will greatly reduce your burden. However, this on its own will not be enough to enable the carer to be protected from stress. Over the years, Penny has found it essential for there to be a Carer's New Project. This is an entirely new activity that is chosen by the main carer and taken forward by them in some way, however slowly. It is a pleasurable pastime that has come about as a result of becoming involved in SPECALCARE but at the same time has nothing whatsoever to do with dementia. The Project may be associated with a previous interest or enthusiasm: one carer recently chose miniature painting, having been an artist for years but never having had the time to study this particular skill. It may, on the other hand, be something entirely unconnected with previous activities: one carer learnt to use a computer, and another, much to Penny's dismay, announced that she had always wanted to learn to ride a horse – she was over 70. Interestingly, when Penny said that nothing was too wacky to be included on the initial list of possibilities, the carer began to have doubts, and these became more concrete when Penny suggested the Tipping Point might be when *the carer* had had a certain number of falls. She eventually decided to take up Fair Isle Knitting instead.

The Carer's New Project has two main purposes: the first is to provide something positive and concrete that has arisen from the encounter with dementia through SPECAL. This provides a point of interest apart from the dementia itself, while being in some sense directly associated with it. The second purpose is to ensure that the carer is gradually developing a new area of their life as the client's dependency on them is progressively reduced via an increasingly skilled care team. There is clear evidence that the guilt so often cited by carers is vastly reduced by the application of a Profile for the client's care running in parallel with the pursuit of a new interest by the carer. We have instances of carers creating a new social network for themselves that is independent of the client and should, ideally, begin to be developed as soon as possible after the client's diagnosis.

In the vast majority of cases there will come a time when it will no longer be best for the client to be cared for at home. The Carer's New Project really comes into its own in helping to avoid a vacuum if and when the client moves out of the family home. This time may lie well ahead in the future, but now is the right moment to be planning for it – and how to do so, ensuring 24-hour wraparound care, is explained in Part Three.

TROUBLESHOOTING

'I am not enthusiastic about forming a team, because I don't want to involve friends and neighbours with my caring problems. Should I just wait and see who comes forward?'
It is important to realise how much people like to help in small ways, and how often they feel excluded by the carer. Friends and neighbours just need to know that they are important, and that they can make a positive contribution just by understanding what SPECALSENSE is all about.

'My children have enough problems of their own, without being given extra worries of helping as part of my team. I feel I should let them get on with their own lives. Surely this is right?'
Your children are already emotionally involved, and probably far

more than you realise. As with the friends and neighbours, but much more so, most family members would prefer to know that they are helping you rather than feel that they are of little value. At Burford, over the years we have been amazed at the way in which whole families come together, both emotionally and in a practical way, once the spotlight is turned to the single focus of the client's well-being. Many families report that they are more 'in tune' with each other as a family than ever before, once they start working together to help the carer develop the Profile.

Part Three

PLANNING FOR THE FUTURE

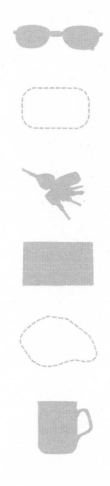

Introduction

Many carers have an absolute horror of their client entering a nursing home and that is not just because of the phenomenal expense. The dread is of dumping their beloved one in an uncaring, bewildering, impersonal environment. It is worth reflecting on the way in which dog owners with ageing pooches put off the awful day when their cherished canine has to be taken to the vet to be put down. Somehow, 'today' never seems to be the right time, although the poor thing is obviously in great discomfort and pain. Similarly, too many carers feel unable to consider the client's point of view, caught up as they are with an unbearable sense of guilt and self-doubt.

Penny Garner could not disagree more strongly with this perception. Her experience over numerous years has enabled her to prove to the carer's satisfaction that there comes a stage in almost every case where it is absolutely imperative for the *client's* well-being that they move to a nursing home. Once the Care Profile is designed and brought into use, and the client's dementia has reached a certain stage (assessed in terms of how few new facts are being stored), the client will benefit hugely by spending time in the company of their peers – other people with dementia.

There is another, equally important but sometimes forgotten, reason for viewing the planning of the transition to a nursing home as a natural investment in the future rather than a collapse of the past: every carer has a life of their own to lead and this becomes increasingly difficult while running a private nursing home for one person in the family home.

A sound reason for being prepared for the transition as soon as possible after diagnosis (which is not the same as actually making the move – far from it), is that a crisis could occur at any time. This is nothing to do with dementia, but rather a general statement applicable to any of us. We can all fall ill, and dementia carers and dementia clients are no exception.

SPECAL talks of a Tipping Point. This is not the point at which the client gets tipped into a nursing home, nor is it when the carer's sanity finally tips into oblivion. The Tipping Point is the one at which the balance of benefits to the client of remaining at home is just beginning to tip in favour of moving. This is the point, well ahead of major problems (ruling out sudden unforeseen crises), when the family need to change gear and prepare for a smooth move. It may be that the client has physical disabilities that mean that professional help with lifting and toileting is required. Even if the client needs none of these aids, there comes a point when their best interests will be better served by a move from the family home.

Penny maintains that clients in the later stages of dementia whose SPECALCARE is well developed find the presence of other people with dementia very good company. While their socialising may not make a lot of sense to an untrained outsider, they often manage to provide each other with just the right level of companionship. They do not disturb each other's sense of the situation in which they find themselves. A client is soon feeling at home in a 'hotel' where they have a bed for the night, prior to going on home the next day or so. Carers find it difficult to imagine, until they experience it for themselves, the ease with which the client can adapt to a temporary hotel environment, and how much more sense this setting makes to them than continually trying to fathom out why they feel so alien at home.

Because there is such a strong tendency for carers to blank out the issue of nursing home selection, they are liable not to realise when the Tipping Point has been reached. All too often, they only acknowledge any need for action when a tragedy happens, like a client's fall or their own mental or physical health beginning to crack. Without having made any plans, the transition to a nursing home becomes an enforced and rushed event which compromises choice and often destroys the client's well-being.

For these reasons, Penny insists that every family visits several prospective homes as soon as practicable following the diagnosis of dementia, even if the illness is at a relatively early stage. A suitable home must be identified and agreed between the key family members, and a relationship established with the home's manager, even though a place may not be required for a considerable time into the future. On top of that, every carer needs to have identified in advance what they would regard as their specific Tipping Point. They also need to draw up a provisional plan for making a future transition to the nursing home as part of the completed Care Profile. The various steps that are entailed in actually making the move also need to be considered, along with the possibility of a period in hospital on the way if a physical ailment should arise to trigger the move.

CHAPTER TWELVE

Find your Tipping Point and Choose a Nursing Home

FIND YOUR TIPPING POINT

Looking for this probably seems like the very last thing you want to do right now – like reviewing your bank statements after you have gone bankrupt – it's too depressing on top of all the other worries that beset you. But failure to identify your Tipping Point right now puts at risk all the work you have done in reading this book and setting up wraparound care. Now is the moment to face up to the reality that providing care will undoubtedly become too much for you one day. However upsetting or seemingly depressing, you absolutely have to apply your mind to establishing a Tipping Point for the future, writing it on a special piece of paper which you then keep safely in the back of your drawer. This is your insurance policy for the future, a safety valve, a fallback position and a source of calm.

What you are looking for is the situation where you would say to yourself, 'This is absurd. I just cannot go on like this.' To find it, ask yourself what have been the worst scenarios you have encountered in the last few weeks in relation to providing care for your client. Write down your selection, including any that have happened only once, and then put them in order of awfulness. Penny Garner advocates making a beeline for one-off ghastly events, the ones you would prefer to be putting right out of your mind. Now take the worst one and decide how many times it would need to happen within a given time frame for you to reach that 'this is absurd' moment – something like 'I would reach the Tipping Point if this happened twice in a week' or 'once a fortnight', a frequency within a time scale.

For one wife caring for her husband, it was a question of how much missed sleep could be tolerated. He was liable to stay up late and it was impossible to get him to bed earlier. While he could sleep in until ten or eleven, she had to get up earlier than that to organise the house and fulfil other commitments. Pressed to quantify the problem, she felt she could cope with late nights once a week but that twice a week would send her over the cliff of exhaustion.

In another case it was being unable to get the client upstairs to bed. And in another, one kettle too many boiling dry and almost setting the house alight. A daughter who lived with her mother listed several worst moments, including having found her mother slumped on the floor in terrible pain one morning having fallen out of bed and damaged her ankle. Yet the daughter told Penny that her list contained nothing that she felt was too difficult to cope with, however often it might occur. Only when pressed by Penny to explore further could the daughter nail down what would tip her over the edge. Her mother had fallen asleep on the loo twice, risking a dangerous fall in a very confined space and with a locked door. Eventually, it was decided that if she were to find her mother asleep on the loo twice in one week, the daughter would accept the need for a nursing home.

Penny has encouraged countless carers to do just what they

don't want to do – explore those worst-case scenarios which everyone would so much rather ignore.

In a few cases, you may find that in doing this exercise you have already passed the Tipping Point. One daughter who did not live with her mother described being woken in the middle of the night by telephone calls. Her mother would be having a panic attack, screaming for help and unable to hear her daughter's words of reassurance because she was so hard of hearing. The daughter reflected that 'My mother wants someone there right now, but I cannot be there and every time it happens I think "this can't go on".' Putting a limit of once a week for this to happen as being just about acceptable, she then realised with a shock that it was already happening more than that. In identifying that the Tipping Point had been passed she said 'Actually, it's a great relief to realise that this has got to end *for her good*. In the past I have always felt guilty when considering a nursing home, liable to castigate myself for just wanting to bundle the old ratbag off and get her out of the way.' Like plenty of other offspring and not a few spouses, this daughter was well aware that she felt considerable hostility towards her mother dating back to childhood. In considering the problem calmly and objectively, she was able to see beyond the inevitable emotions that this charged issue can so often raise.

Now that you have sorted the Tipping Point, you need to take the next step: deciding on the nursing home of the family's choice.

CHOOSE A NURSING HOME

Penny offers 12 criteria by which to evaluate a potential home for a client (see pages 227–30). One of these is a willingness on the part of any home to take an interest in the work you are doing. In the past Penny would suggest that the carer provide the home under consideration with a SPECAL leaflet, to give them a flavour of the approach. One carer reported that the home she was considering took one look at the front cover, handed it back without reading it, and said, 'Oh, we do that sort of thing ourselves when the resident first moves in.' Now you will be able to run the same acid test for yourself by passing over this book for perusal and seeing what happens.

Most homes train their staff in person-centred care and are likely to be interested in anything that will help the resident move in with ease. You will be able to explain about a document called the 'SPECAL Passport' that you will prepare ahead of the move and share with the home.[10] The Passport is created out of a distillation of all the knowledge about the client that you have gleaned since those early days when you first developed the Profile. The Passport is a single sheet of paper that lists six questions and provides the answers, as follows:

CORE QUESTION: What do I need to know in order to get alongside this person without relying on their recall of any information relating to the recent past?

The succeeding five questions and their individual answers, provide the overall answer to this core question.

---

[10] Several key documents now used by SPECAL during the client's nursing home transition were originally developed in collaboration with the nursing staff at Burford Hospital during the 1990s. See Johns, C. [ed.], 1994, 'The Burford NDU Model: Caring in Practice', Oxford: Blackwell Scientific Publications.

Question 1. Who is this person?

In fact, the answer to this is who this person *used* to be, especially the roles they enjoyed occupying, socially and professionally. The answer is in the Primary Theme and is mostly concerned with carefully chosen details of the client's personality and mannerisms.

Question 2: What key questions am I likely to be asked by this person and what answers should I give?

The answer provides the questions and answers that have been SPOTted – the repetitive issues and topics that you have learned to love, often closely linked to the Primary Theme.

Question 3: What health reason (apart from dementia) is there for this person to be in a care setting?

This is the Health Theme.

Question 4: What are the crucial props associated with the promotion of well-being?

This includes all the physical props or catchphrases you have identified, including those for the Primary Theme.

Question 5: What is the bottom-line strategy if this person does not feel comfortable and wishes to leave?

This is the Altruistic Trigger, the failsafe phrase which will prevent the client from acting dangerously.

What other frequently asked questions, with tried and tested answers, are there?

A typical Passport is shown opposite:

SPECAL Passport

CORE QUESTION: *What do I need to know in order to get alongside this person without relying on their recall of any information relating to the recent past?*

Who is this person?
Tony is a retired scriptwriter who is familiar with many aspects of broadcasting. He is a person with a developed sense of gallantry to others, and a smile that intermittently lights up his face and then slowly fades away, only to return seconds later. He has a keen but gentle wit, often against himself and never unkind. He needs time to deliver his lines. His ready conversation often moves seamlessly to and fro between literature and music, in a delightfully engaging way. He loves sitting quietly listening to music.

What key questions am I likely to be asked by this person and what answers should I give?
– Where's my wife/June? (answer: *June is sorting her parents out*)
– Where's Sophie/Hannah? (answer: *In London*)
– Where's Wally? (answer: *Wally's gone out for a walk*)
– Where am I? (answer: *This is a SPECAL hotel*)
– What's all that noise? (answer: *They must be rehearsing their lines*)
– Where's my money? (answer: *In the bank*)
– How much money have I got? (answer: *Plenty/lots*)
– Where's my wallet? (answer: *June is bringing it in*)
– What does it cost? (answer: *It's all paid for – by June*)
Catch-all answers that often work for many questions are: 'I will go and find out' and 'We must ask June.'

What health reason (apart from dementia) is there for this person to be in a care setting?
Tony had a gallstone operation many years ago and can recall a hilarious themed party he went to soon afterwards, given by a medical friend. Tony went as a Cossack with a white frilly shirt. His wound suppurated, the shirt turned red in the front and he appeared to be a Cossack who had been in a fight! The doctor had to take him upstairs and wind a huge bandage round his middle. Everyone found this highly entertaining, including Tony and June, and 'gallstones' has remained as a potential health need to be addressed.

What are the crucial props associated with the promotion of well-being?
The phrase 'in sync'. The book of complete works of Lewis Carroll. 'The Hunting of the Snark'. Torch. Music CD (Debussy). His notebook and pencil.

What is the bottom-line strategy if this person does not feel comfortable and wishes to leave?
The phrase 'June would be really worried.'

Regarding which nursing home you choose, as already noted, it is essential that the head of the home who is going to be taking over the day-to-day coordination of care from you has read this book. Beyond that, Penny suggests going to visit at least four prospective homes before you make your final decision and then visiting the preferred home at least once more to fix it in your mind. Once you have made the final choice, you put the client's name down as someone who is on their list, albeit that you cannot say when the day will dawn.

On the whole, Penny finds that carers tend to get a feel for whether they think a care home is good or not very quickly and that it is a very personal decision, with much variability as to what is most important. Just as house buyers have instant and powerful responses when shown round a potential new house, so too, it would seem, with nursing homes. Penny recalls wondering how on earth she would ever be able to decide which school they should choose for her eldest daughter Clare. When she asked an older friend for advice they said, 'When you're sitting listening to the headmistress telling you about the school, imagine that it is very late at night and you have a huge concern about Clare. Can you see yourself having the courage to pick up the phone and possibly wake this person up? If so, it's probably the right school!'

Carers usually find it helpful to consider all the issues listed below. For each of the 12 criteria which follow, give a cross or a tick. In asking these questions, Penny advocates being in a relaxed but observant mode. After all, you really don't know much about any of these homes, so don't visit as a suspicious, dubious relative, but take it all in. You will find it easier to absorb the atmosphere if you take someone with you so that you have someone to debrief with afterwards. Provided you come across as friendly, the staff will not become defensive and you are more likely to get a fair picture as to what life in that home is all about.

1. Is it readily accessible to the main carer from the family home?

It is useful if the nursing home is reasonably close, as the family will need to be available to shadow the care in the home during the initial transition. However it should not be next door either, or the carer may find it difficult to 'let go'. Once the client is completely settled in, the carer will only need to visit once a week from the point of view of sustaining client well-being, although the carer may wish to visit more often for other reasons (see below for further explanation of this).

2. Does it provide an attractive atmosphere?

The best way to decide is by asking yourself, 'Would I like to live there if I were the client?'

3. Does it have an accessible, secure garden, with two ways of getting into it from the building?

Two entrances mean that the person can wander out on their own, and anyone wanting to join them or encourage them back in, can walk outside by the other door and meet the client rather than have to chase after them. Two points of access to any secure garden is a bonus for dementia care.

4. Does it have an acceptable level of physical/emotional risk?

The best way to judge this is to ask, 'Would it feel free, safe, comfortable and homely to the client?'

5. Are there adequate opportunities for personal choice?

For example, is the programme of daily activities optional? Is there a 'quiet room' so the client can get some peace from the noise of other clients? How much choice of seating areas, including little nooks, could you choose from when visiting the client?

6. Is there easy access to common areas for socialising?

Homes are generally too isolating, and the person with dementia needs other people around for orientation. Shared rooms and dormitories are brilliant but sadly, at the moment, have been completely phased out of nursing homes. If left to their own devices without other people around, clients can easily lose their sense of time and place. Remember that a person with dementia should never be left entirely alone – they always need shadowing. In Dorothy's case, for example, being in places where there are no other people would have made her wonder if she had missed her flight. Alice would feel that her Bridge Club had been disbanded. It is far easier to provide a non-threatening context for a group of people than it is to explain solitary confinement in a chic private room with en suite facilities.

7. Will you be able to afford it for three years?

Penny believes that in the later stages of dementia, if the transition has been seamlessly achieved, a move to a less expensive home will not pose a problem after three years of green in the nursing home of choice. The client's default position by then is consolidated as green and will stay that way provided any move is carried out according to the template of the first.

8. What is the home's approach to care planning?

It's worth asking to see an example of a care plan, as it will give you some idea of how much emphasis is on physical care and how much on other more esoteric areas of life. If the plan majors on bowel movements, say 'how wonderful' and ask if there's anything else – act the innocent and get the maximum information.

9. What sounds can be heard in the background? Are they pleasant or otherwise?

Take a moment, maybe stand by a window, close your eyes and listen. Can you hear the birds singing? On your second visit you might try dozing off in a chair, your eyes shut. What impression do you gain of the environment? The sounds that you hear can tell you a great deal, and they are, in a sense, the background music of the home. If you hear a strange noise from time to time, what acceptable explanation can you find to give the client if they ask?

10. What is the attitude towards visitors or pets – are there any restrictions regarding visiting times, numbers of visitors, presence/absence of animals?

It is interesting to see how the manager of the home reacts to the idea of bringing a dog – 'good heavens no' is one thing, 'alas, not possible' is another. Some homes are actually quite happy with cats and goldfish.

11. What is the attitude/response to SPECAL ideas?

You might try out one of the three commandments on them – 'I have found it's best not to ask him/her questions. What do you find?'

12. What is the attitude towards medication? Do they see it as a way of silencing or immobilising difficult people?

Remember to appear naïve when asking about it – 'I don't quite understand what all this business with drugs is about. When do you generally find they need to be given?' In terms of anti-dementia drugs, it is interesting that the SPECAL approach was developed in the days when these drugs were not yet available, and that they are unnecessary for SPECALCARE.

In most cases, Penny finds that carers do not have much trouble choosing between different homes. However, in the event of not being able to decide, you can give a score out of 5 for each of these criteria and tot up which has the highest. While not a definitive solution, it may help to swing the decision one way or the other.

Having organised a home, there is one last preparatory step to be taken: arming yourself with a plan for the actual transition to the nursing home. The best way to explain this is to leap forward to the advice Penny offers for actually making that transition.

The next chapter explains how to transfer your managerial role to the nursing home without putting your client at risk of reds. It will repay those readers who have not yet reached their Tipping Point to read this as well because it will explain where the work as a carer is ultimately leading and how to prepare a plan for the move.

CHAPTER THIRTEEN

Prepare a Transitional Care Plan for Making the Move

Given that you are going to feel pretty hard-pressed when you reach the Tipping Point, it is very helpful to have already worked out as many as possible of the practicalities and other things for the move, setting them out in your notebook. Heaven forefend, but something could always happen to you, leaving your other care team members unsure what to do. Also, when the time for the move does come, you will want to ensure that everyone is singing from the same hymn sheet and the transitional care plan is that sheet: a written statement that can be handed to everyone involved.

While not all the details of the plan can be identified at this stage, many of them can be set down, leaving it until later to mark in the details. Eventually, you will need to set out the following and circulate copies to everyone concerned:

- The plan you have for dealing with client questions arising from visiting the nursing home, from the car park onwards.
- The name and number of the key worker at the nursing home.

- Names and contact numbers of the people who will be on the rota for an initial 72-hour period of intensive support.
- A timetable for the move.

There is one other eventuality which needs considering for a comprehensive SPECAL plan: hospital admissions.

HOSPITAL ADMISSIONS

Given that the client is elderly, there is a high likelihood that at some point they will have to spend one or more nights in hospital. In some cases, it may be that the transition to the nursing home will be from hospital, if physical illness has caused the Tipping Point to be passed.

It will be extremely difficult, if not impossible, to protect your client from any red if they are admitted to hospital. One reason is that the nursing staff often change too frequently for you to be able to explain the Passport to them, another is that they may be simply too busy to take it on board. A further problem is that visiting hours limit how much time you can spend there. For these reasons, you need to set up a rota to visit at all hours possible and you may well find that you have to use the 'getting from red to green' tool more than once.

One useful tip is that all wards will have a care plan for your client. If you can gain the attention of the chief nurse and if you select a single key care strategy, you can ask that it be added to the care plan. If that happens, all nurses who are on duty will be expected to implement it. However, the strategy has to be something that can be done with no SPECAL training. For example, one carer had developed a highly effective technique for getting their client to take pills. Once it was explained and demonstrated to the chief nurse, it was helpfully incorporated into the care plan. Another example was a client who would only eat meals if sitting on the edge of the bed. So long as the proposals are highly practical and simple, you should be able to get at least one written in.

But overall, hospital admissions are liable to create a lot of red and the sooner you can get your client moved to a care home, the better, once their physical condition has stabilised.

MAKING THE MOVE

It is time for you to hand over to a care setting where the carers work in shifts – it is simply neither sensible nor desirable for a single home carer to cope with the physical demands any longer. However, it is vital that the Care Profile continues to be employed if the client is to stay away from reds; indeed, it is a key feature of SPECALCARE that it is designed to be transferable and wraparound in a formal care setting.

You have already identified a nursing home with a manager who has read or will read this book, and now that the time for transition has come, you go and visit them on your own. You talk through the Care Profile and the Passport alongside their own admission and assessment paperwork so that you are both happy with the dovetailing which is needed. The manager will then be in a good position to ensure that all staff read the Passport and understand its significance.

The first step is to arrange to make at least two or three visits to the home with the client on successive days before the day of the move. You also need to have another member of the family or a friend to help, by being already installed in the home when you arrive with the client each day. This creates a ready-made party for you and the client to join. The purpose of the visits is to SPOT the client's reaction to the setting, to troubleshoot any obvious problems, to develop conversational routines that fit the new setting, and to familiarise the staff with these once they have become established. In the case of Tony, the client whose Passport was described in Chapter 12, he was enjoying a cup of coffee on one of the initial visits when one of the other clients at the home began screeching in an alarming fashion: 'Help, help, aaaaaagh!' Tony was really thrown, and everyone stiffened wondering what to say. Quick-thinking saved the day. 'Quite a rehearsal!' Penny Garner commented to him, raising her eyebrows. Tony smiled and nodded, completely relaxed. Since his Primary Theme concerned the theatre, this was a completely acceptable explanation for the noise and any other untoward happening that subsequently occurred.

Another reason for the visits is to establish some useful routines and rituals based on the client's lead in providing conversational patter that is found to work. These give everyone confidence as the new routines build up. Although the client is unlikely to be storing many facts, they are always storing feelings. By spending short periods of time there happily, they will start storing positive feelings about being there. The staff will also become more familiar with the client.

To make these visits you use the same techniques as you would make for any other journey. You will have a well-established reason for leaving the house together, making use of the we-relationship, be it to go to the golf club, to the shops or to see a friend. However, this time you will need to have planned in considerable detail the potential problems you may encounter when the car comes to a halt in the nursing home car park. The question may come from the client, 'Why have we stopped here?' You need an acceptable reason that will probably relate to their Primary Theme and will incorporate a cup of tea in the nursing home. If the theme is golf, you might reply, 'We've come to see someone who can't play golf because of an injury' or if the theme is Bridge, it might be, 'There's someone here who wants to learn about Bridge.' Whatever you settle on, as ever, it must be authentic and you will need to have identified ways in which you will be able to develop it once inside the home. As usual, you will have any travelling props with you, along with your armoury of gestures and key phrases.

Having written down your answer to the initial question – 'Why have you stopped in this car park?' – you need further answers prepared for likely subsidiary questions. If you are going down the injured golfer road, you need some details of who they are which plug into the theme to answer the question, 'Who is it that is injured?' You may need there to be someone in the home who connects to this, maybe someone with a bad back. If you are playing the Bridge card, you may need an answer to questions such as, 'Is this a Bridge Club?' and, 'I don't remember coming here before.' You may need to reference someone who is prepared to show an interest in the client's expertise in the area of the Primary Theme, using well-established verbal ping-pong routines.

Once inside the home, apart from looking for potential pitfalls, you need to ensure that the other family member (or perhaps a friend) is already installed in the sitting room ready to welcome you both. You settle down for a cup of tea and then you need to use the usual Explanations for Departure and Absence. You then shadow from a distance. You may notice things to draw to the attention of the key worker or to other staff members. Without being annoying or fussy, take every chance just to help the staff understand what works with the client, making connections to the Passport which all of them will have seen. You either return to pick up the client and go home together, or you may prefer to go home ahead and let the client return home with the other family member or friend. You then re-run the same procedure on at least two consecutive days.

On the day of the move, proceed in exactly the same way as on previous days. The nursing home will probably try to persuade you to come around midday but it is much better to negotiate that you arrive with the client in the late afternoon shortly before the evening meal. There will have been no conversation about spending the night, and any luggage will have been sent on in advance. You have the tea party as on previous visits, and you, the main carer, then withdraw from the client's company using your Explanation for Departure as before. The other family member (or a member of the staff) gradually introduces the idea of having supper and spending the night in such a way that the client will assume it was the plan all along. Precisely how they do so depends on the Primary or Health Theme but it will entail much use of a combination of Themes, Explanations and the Altruistic Trigger. Negotiations will only be around the idea of a single night's stay, when the idea is first introduced to the client. The inference may be that this is a hotel from which golf might take place. Alternatively, it could be that they have come into a hospital for a routine check up just for the night. Whatever the narrative, you remain on site, but if possible out of sight, until they are bedded down and asleep. Be constantly on alert for amber and ready to support the staff. For example, one client was just being settled into their room when a staff member knocked on the door and asked, 'What would you like for breakfast?' Since the matter of spending the night had not yet been introduced, the client said, 'No thanks, I won't be needing any breakfast, I'm not staying here.' It took some time for the carer to recover the situation, testing every element of the Care Profile to the absolute limit – from the Primary Theme via the Health

Theme all the way to the last resort of the Altruistic Trigger (which happily and predictably proved its worth).

Prior to embarking on any of this you will have constructed a rota from your core team players to ensure that someone is on call at all times for the first 72 hours of the client's stay. Ideally, during this time, the client should have no waking hours when there is not someone from the core team of family carers at the nursing home. While incredibly gruelling for all concerned, it is absolutely critical that the client's initial experience of the home is as green as possible. The effort expended at this point will be an invaluable investment in the future well-being of both client and carer and will save everyone enormous amounts of time and trouble in the longer term. Hence, you need to be there when the client wakes up on the first morning and have someone else to take over so you can get a break that day. This needs to be kept up continuously, ensuring that the client remains in green and, wherever possible, gently explaining to staff members with whom there is contact how to apply the Passport.

If all goes smoothly, from the fourth day onwards there need only be a daily visit. This visit should be at the time identified as the most problematic one during the initial 72-hour period. It might be waking or bedtime, it might be a mealtime. Whatever it is, there needs to be someone there to shadow and help the staff to find the best solution. Again, if all goes smoothly, after anything from a week later up to a few weeks, it should become possible for the visits to be reduced to every other day, then every third day, then only once weekly. With this degree of monitoring, it should be possible to get the client happily green at the home. Although their conversations with the other clients may make no sense to outsiders, there is plenty to talk about, prompting positive feelings. Because there is shift work, the client no longer depends on an exhausted or stressed carer, and the staff will become increasingly tuned in to them with the help of their Passport.

The scene is set for sustained well-being but it is not realistic to assume that all will go 100 per cent smoothly the entire time. It is inevitable that setbacks will occasionally occur. The way we deal with setbacks is to take a close look at how the potentially red situation is arising, and draft a risk management plan to ensure that an amber does not become a red. This plan identifies the risk, with a primary focus on the emotional element, sets out one or more strategic interventions, and considers the implications for staff members, other residents, family or friends.

RISK MANAGEMENT STRATEGY

There are emotional as well as physical aspects to risk, and it is important to make the emotional aspect the primary consideration for the SPECAL client, on the basis that the physical implications then become relatively easy to accommodate. The reverse approach to risk management has been shown to be much less effective in promoting a continuity of acceptable experience for the client.

Where a client's behaviour is defined as being high risk, either to themselves or others, SPECAL identifies the area of risk and introduces something (an activity, or a place, or a person) that will act as the agent for change. The minimum amount of shadowing needed in order to monitor the management strategy using SPOT is also identified.

Before the strategy is implemented, the issues are discussed either individually or collectively with everyone concerned, to ensure that they are understood.

A typical risk management strategy sheet is set out overleaf.[11] It relates to the case history of Michael and Valerie which follows this chapter.

It is important that there are weekly visits from the carer or a member of the core team from home care, to check that the green is still persisting and to keep an eye out for physical illnesses that the staff may not pick up, as well as fulfilling the carer's need to spend time with the person they love. Penny's experience with Dorothy taught her that it is vital to pop in regularly and make an emotional connection to ensure the client is okay. It is important to remind yourself who this older person would have been if they did not have dementia: they would, in any case, have grown more frail with age, spending increasing amounts of time asleep or in an inward-looking frame of mind, focusing on their inner life. Penny believes this was her mother's principal state of mind for much of her waking life in her later years. Penny found she usually only needed to touch her mother's hand or make a familiar gesture or use some other way to get her attention, and then a sparkle of eye-contact would occur. Invisible to outsiders, it is like a bolt of electricity, a moment in which the carer can see that the person they love is still there, that emotionally they are still the same person they always were; that there is a moment of recognition from the client at a 'feelings' level, even if – in the later stages of dementia – they may have no idea what your name is. They recognise you as friend, not foe.

[11] For further background to the development of this strategy, see Johns, C. [ed.], 1994, 'The Burford NDU Model: Caring in Practice', Oxford: Blackwell Scientific Publications.

Risk Management Strategy

NAME OF CLIENT: VALERIE
DATE: January 2008
Identified risk: That Valerie will feel disempowered if she is restrained by other people when she chooses to move around the home without assistance.

Background:
Valerie was recently admitted to Park House from hospital, following a fall at home. Valerie sustained a leg fracture and is in plaster. Guidance from the hospital is to avoid weight-bearing at present. Valerie sees no reason to restrict her movements around Park House and strongly resents interference from staff when she chooses to walk about. Valerie has an independent nature and is used to calling the shots in her own home. Valerie has expressed her wish to move about without obstruction from others using a degree of physical violence towards anyone getting in her way. Valerie has expressed her wish to use a Zimmer frame by helping herself to one belonging to another resident, and this has produced a potentially explosive situation in which staff have to intervene.

The primary focus is to manage the emotional risk that Valerie's sense of well-being will be compromised. Provided this is satisfactorily addressed, the physical risk that Valerie's rehabilitation programme will be compromised can then be addressed. Physical restraint of Valerie is considered only as a last resort.

Strategy:
- Staff will allocate a Zimmer frame to Valerie. This will be kept near to hand and offered to Valerie if she indicates a wish to move about.
- If Valerie is seen moving around with a Zimmer, she will be shadowed with a view to increasing the likelihood that she will wish to sit down for a therapeutic rest on her travels.
- Wherever Valerie is, she should be within easy reach of a book about horses or flowers, or a newspaper, preferably the *Racing Post*.
- If Valerie heads for anyone else's Zimmer she is to be offered her own before the other one is removed from her.

Implications for others:
Staff need to be aware of situations where Valerie may feel a sense of ownership of other people's Zimmer frames, and to ensure that a spare Zimmer for Valerie is available.

Comments:
Staff will need to give themselves consent to place Valerie's emotional risk ahead of her physical risk, and to understand the rationale for this (possibly unusual) strategy.

On every one of the four occasions that Penny could not make this contact, she realised that Dorothy was ill with an infection which needed appropriate medication. If the lack of contact is not due to physical illness, and it is clear that the client is experiencing red, use the 'getting from red to green' solution (see Chapter 6 – get alongside them with the 'we' club, help to orientate them, then flip back to the present day). You should obviously not leave until green is re-established. Once restored, the green should endure, although in extreme cases it may be necessary to reinstate the 72-hour rota again.

Once the client has settled in and is embedded securely in green, it is time to restore the friends and family visitors who were in contact with the client before the move to the nursing home. These will all be familiar with the Passport and will only need a set of basic guidelines to remind them of the key aspects of visiting, and to highlight the need to link with the main carer after their visit. Penny recommends that the main carer accompanies each visitor on their first visit to the home so that everyone's confidence is maintained throughout the visit.

Overleaf is a typical example of a guideline sheet for inducted visitors which has proved its worth.

Guidelines For Visitors To Tony At Bluebell Court

Beforehand, please:
- Tell June when you plan to visit.
- Visit on your own (only one visitor at a time).
- Be prepared to provide June with a few notes and quotes after your visit.

On arrival at Bluebell Court, please:
- Leave your hat and coat on the way in.
- Carry a paper/book/sewing, etc., so that you don't appear to be 'visiting Tony' in any formal, pre-planned fashion.
- Arrive in the room as if you are living just along the corridor and have just caught sight of Tony as you're passing.
- [If Tony is awake and meets your gaze] Smile and greet him as if he has just made your day – 'How *nice* to see you!' and wander in.
- [If Tony is asleep] Slide into a chair, read your newspaper or whatever, and wait for him to wake up and take in your presence – then when he meets your gaze smile and greet him as above.
- Don't bring the outside world into the room – you both share the same world in that you are two people sitting together, interested in literature and music.
- Use the phrase 'in sync' at an appropriate moment, to indicate how 'together' you are in your view of the world.
- Assume that you are seen as a fellow resident by Tony, unless he makes it clear that he is aware that you are coming in from the outside world.
- Stop talking as soon as Tony starts.
- Don't ask questions.
- When replying to Tony's questions, give only one piece of information and embed it in 'good news'.
- When everything is going well, and before either of you tire, murmur about needing to go to the bathroom (or similar), and wander out of the room.
- Tell a member of staff that you are leaving.
- Jot down a few quotes or questions to pass on to June.

It is difficult for carers to believe that the transition will bring about a state of permanent ease for the client and that the suspension of anxious questioning will finally be completed. However, after helping many families over the years, SPECAL knows that the application of the Passport really works, seamlessly. Once the client is settled in, everyone can relax.

TROUBLESHOOTING

'What should I do if the nursing home staff seem resistant to the idea of SPECALSENSE?'

It is quite understandable for professionals to be concerned, or even sceptical, about what may seem to them an entirely new and nonsensical way of approaching dementia. Make an appointment and explain to them that homes that have already been involved with SPECAL families have found the experience cost-effective and rewarding in terms of higher staff morale. There are specific courses available for professionals, enabling them to increase their knowledge, skills and experience and to relate this to the specific case of your own client in a dynamic way.

Case History: The Story of Michael and Valerie, Illustrating SPECALCARE from Beginning to End

This section is included in order to illustrate to you the typical trials and tribulations that carers pass through on their way to creating wraparound care. Hopefully, it will give you confidence that you can make SPECALSENSE work in your case.

Penny Garner was sitting in her office at Burford Hospital in 2005. It had been 30 years since her stark meeting in Lymington with her mother Dorothy's GP. It had been 15 years since she first arrived in the hospital clutching an Alzheimer's Society badge. Today she was waiting for Michael who had just attended a SPECAL photograph album presentation. Michael had asked to see her afterwards.

Penny knew quite a bit about him. He lived in Yorkshire and he and his wife Valerie were staying with their very old friend, Rupert, near Burford. Rupert had for many years been a volunteer member of the Friday Group care team and had finally persuaded Michael to come to hear Penny. Valerie had been diagnosed with dementia three years earlier and life for them both was verging on the chaotic.

Rupert had approached Penny several times wanting to know how he might help Michael and Valerie. He knew Michael as a man blessed with a head full of common sense and strong views, and Rupert also knew enough about dementia to realise that Michael was rapidly becoming expert at unwittingly making a difficult situation almost unmanageable at home. He could see clearly what was going on every time Michael and Valerie came to stay. Penny had repeatedly advised Rupert to get Michael to a photograph album presentation and today, at long last, this had been achieved.

Penny also knew that Michael and Valerie had no children of their own, but that Valerie had had two sons by her first marriage. Michael had become a devoted and dutiful stepfather to Stephen and Peter, and been deeply distressed when Stephen died at a tragically young age. Peter now lived close to the family home in Yorkshire and shared Valerie's interest in breeding thoroughbred racehorses. Valerie's finest equestrian hour had been when her homebred Bounding Bandit won a major cup. Michael shared this passion and they had a deep commitment to each other.

Penny looked up as Michael was ushered in. They shook hands and exchanged the usual pleasantries. As they chatted on, he regaled her with a series of stories to show her how crazy Valerie had become, tales of irrational behaviour and daily arguments. There was a desperate tone to his voice. He explained that he loved his wife and was determined to keep her at home, would never 'put her away'. He wanted to know how to persuade her to alter her behaviour. Penny's heart was rapidly sinking. Michael reminded her of her father Sam, who never understood the need to change his own ways, rather than trying to get his wife to change. Unless Penny could make a serious impact on this man, the situation in Yorkshire would get worse and worse. He and Valerie were out of reach of the Friday Group and the new carer training programme, and for the umpteenth time she wished that someone had written a book about SPECAL that she could give to Michael to take back with him to Yorkshire. But this was 2005 and there was no such book.

As the meeting's end approached she had a choice: confine herself to a few encouraging words – that she knew wouldn't change the long-term situation at all – or challenge Michael head-on, and hope for the best. She had never directly challenged Sam in the old days, but had at least been able to take over responsibility for Dorothy's care herself. She had no such option in Valerie's case, whose future happiness seemed to depend on what happened there in that room. Taking a deep breath, she weighed in.

She explained firmly that there was no need to give any more examples of the chaos that was reigning in Yorkshire. If Michael was prepared to follow her instructions carefully, together they could combine their knowledge and skills, and make huge progress. To Penny's relief, Michael immediately wanted to know what he could do. He loved Valerie to bits and would do anything he could for her. His face lit up as he said, 'What do I have to do?'

While there were several wobbles before Michael completely applied himself to the job, eventually, back in Yorkshire, he struck up a telephone and e-mail relationship with Penny to draw on her expertise.

GETTING GOING

Penny asked Michael to follow the three commandments – don't ask questions, learn from Valerie's repetition and never contradict. Small rewards began to trickle in. Michael found that Valerie became less difficult if he avoided cross-examining her and that there were fewer arguments once he stopped disagreeing with her all the time. When Valerie repeated the same story again and again, he learned to limit his response to a smile and one comment, 'You've been so clever about all that.' He recorded in his diary, 'I am trying to be more SPECAL conscious and I think I am being a bit more successful.'

He began to record Valerie's questions and Penny was able to e-mail further guidance. He learned how to follow the threads of Valerie's various bizarre statements, rather than dismissing them as meaningless. He could then have a stab at guessing where her anxiety was coming from. He started to reflect on Valerie's earlier life – those long-ago days that he felt were an eternity away, before the dementia arrived to turn his life upside down. Life with Valerie was still very difficult and Penny knew they desperately needed to find and use Valerie's Primary Theme.

PRIMARY THEME

Michael couldn't really see the point of searching for a past area of expertise for Valerie, pointing out that she didn't do much these days. Penny persisted and asked him to provide some ideas of what he felt might have been a passion in Valerie's life. His reply began, 'Well, there's me, of course, and then I suppose, apart from that, there might be . . .'

Michael's list eventually covered interior decorating, colour schemes, dogs, horses and buying and selling antiques. The interior decorating seemed to be the most likely candidate, as it dated back to the time of Valerie's first marriage. Under instructions from Penny,

Michael tried admiring a piece of furniture that was Valerie's particular favourite. She chatted away, even beginning to smile again. But when he repeated the routine it didn't hold her for long because she was forever turning the conversation to the subject of horses. This was a topic he always tried desperately to avoid because Valerie kept interfering 'absurdly' in the way the horses were being kept. They were expensive thoroughbreds and Valerie's plans for them now tended to be incredibly wide of the mark. The subject brought out the worst in both Michael and Valerie. 'She loves arguing about anything and especially about the horses. Horses are great ones for routine and Valerie is always changing it. When I point this out Valerie starts an argument. We have three horses in training with the same trainer and each one is co-owned by someone different. She can never remember which is which or who is who and which horse they are involved with. Sometimes when we are off to the races Valerie will say to me, "Why are we selling this horse?" She thinks we are going to a sale.' Michael still found himself 'putting Valerie straight' when it came to anything to do with the horses and wanted to keep right off the subject for his own sanity.

Penny asked Michael to have the courage to explore horses more, not less, with Valerie. She pointed out that they were searching for something Valerie was passionate about and horses really did seem to fit the bill. She asked Michael to track all the horsey quotes, Valerie's views on what decisions should be made about the breeding, breaking, training, whatever, and any questions she was asking. Michael somewhat reluctantly complied and reported that Valerie seemed to imagine that her own horses were running in any race she saw on the TV, and that at night she said she felt very tired because she had been so busy with the horses all day. When he added that in fact Valerie had not seen the horses for over a fortnight, Penny reminded him that where Valerie was concerned feelings were vastly more important than facts. Penny supplied Michael with a set of questions to think about, including what Valerie's finest hour might have been in relation to horses, and back came the story of winning The Cup. That triggered more questions from Penny and gradually a whole vocabulary began to build up. Michael found a video of the famous race and that became a crucial prop to support the Primary Theme of 'Horses'. Penny also asked Michael to try and discover what Valerie's favourite piece of furniture might be, some further information about her two sons, what food she enjoyed (both in terms of eating and cooking), what her favourite clothes were, and so on.

By now Michael was beginning to see that no detail was too trivial to be left unexplored and that all areas of Valerie's past life, however painful, would need to come under the spotlight, including the untimely death of her son Stephen. SPOTting was becoming a very familiar word. However, he was still unhappy with all the focus on horses and not at all clear how this would in any way help to ensure Valerie's lifelong well-being. He often asked, 'What is the point of all this?'

The search for a Primary Theme might still be going on today if it had not been for a name that emerged as part of Michael's answer to one of Penny's culinary questions. Enter Sheila, a person who was to provide invaluable help to SPECAL over the next two years. Sheila was already hugely relied on in a large number of domestic ways by 'The Captain and Mrs T', as she called them, and was now coming in a great deal to help. Penny was quick to realise that Sheila was a star and pressed Michael to get her to Burford, along with his stepson, Peter. Peter was now in charge of the horses, and his name kept cropping up. Their visit to Burford was duly organised and proved a turning point.

Penny recognised in Sheila another Mildred (Dorothy's dedicated cleaning lady), a person with an instinctive and unconditional positive regard for whomever she happened to be with, always finding a charitable interpretation for even the most outrageous behaviour. She could see both sides of any argument and lived out the idea which Penny had heard from Dorothy years before: 'We all have our reasons at the time for what we do, although we may not necessarily say what they are.'

Sheila was a natural SPOTter and more information flowed in. It was she who confirmed that Mrs T's Primary Theme should be to do with horses and within a day of discussing the matter with Penny, was able to report back that 'The Captain' had agreed. There was now a small team of key supporters grouped around Valerie, all with a good basic understanding of the SPECAL approach – Michael, Peter, Sheila and Rupert. SPECAL was there in the background chivvying the whole thing along from Burford. It was time to tackle the Health Theme.

HEALTH THEME

This was not difficult to identify as Valerie had broken many a bone in the course of horse riding. She was currently using a Zimmer frame, which, although she was taking it in her stride (like any horse enthusiast), limited her activities. That was frustrating and the idea of taking care of herself in order to get fully mobile again was an entirely acceptable concept. All Valerie's dependency problems could now focus on her need to get better in order to take charge of the horses and 'taking care not to take things too quickly' was a great recipe for slowing Valerie down in a number of beneficial ways.

For his part, Michael was apprehensive that yet more of a focus on horses in Valerie's life could only mean misery for everyone else, but Penny assured him he must draw heavily on 'carer's courage' and have trust in the SPECAL programme. There was no time to waste and as soon as the two crucial Themes were in place and in use, attention then turned to the various 'Explanations' that were urgently needed, beginning with the Explanation for Departure. 'Take care of the horses' was a phrase that entered the vocabulary book.

EXPLANATION FOR DEPARTURE

Michael explored all sorts of other Explanations for how he needed to be doing something other than keeping Valerie company all the time. It wasn't long before he spotted that if she asked where he was off to when he left the room, and if it happened to be the loo, Valerie couldn't have been less interested and continued to read the *Racing Post*. Penny was delighted. 'That's it! We have it! Don't use anything else from now on. Great!' Michael was incredulous. 'Surely to goodness you're not suggesting I say that *every* time I get up and walk out, even for a few seconds?' Penny was adamant, 'For the time being, yes please, Michael.' Michael never argued with anyone these days and he was soon reporting that he was now 'going off to the loo with monotonous regularity'. Valerie responded in the same matriarchal way, every single time, as he recorded in his diary:

MICHAEL: Sorry – that coffee goes right through me. I must go for a pee.

VALERIE: You had better be quick – we don't want you doing it in your pants.

He reported in astonishment, 'It seems to work!' No sooner was that all sorted out than it was time to identify the next 'Explanation', the Explanation for Absence of the main carer, once they had left the room.

EXPLANATION FOR ABSENCE

The search began for the best answer which Sheila could give to Valerie when asked to explain where Michael was when he was out of sight and going to be missing for more than a couple of minutes. Penny asked Michael to draw up a list of ideas of 'what I might do tomorrow' as topics to discuss with Valerie over morning coffee each day. He had to talk about tomorrow, and *not* today. The list included 'shooting', 'checking the tractor', 'mending the fences', 'moving the horses', and 'gone to see Peter'. All seemed to have some sort of problem attached to them and he noticed that Valerie nearly always responded with ideas about how she would come too. She could come beating with the dogs – end of 'shooting' as an idea. The tractor might be needed to pull the horsebox out of the mud, so she would come to supervise. The fences clearly involved the horses' safety and she was soon expressing ideas about that. It was no good Penny just saying, 'Don't worry, Michael, as long as you agree with her at the time and keep your confidence high it'll be all right.' He still felt very, very apprehensive and was struggling hard.

The solution came when Valerie happened to say to Sheila, as they were chatting in Michael's absence: 'I suppose he's gone farming. That's good.' Sheila could spot the sense of approval in Valerie's voice and her body language was oozing relaxation as her head nodded in quiet satisfaction. Sheila reported back and Valerie's phrase 'He's farming' entered the profiling dictionary. That response was relayed to everyone and attention turned to the third explanation – the Explanation for Presence of a replacement carer.

EXPLANATION FOR PRESENCE

It was clear that there was no need to have any specific explanation as to why Sheila might be hovering about the house during Michael's absence. Valerie made perfectly good sense of Sheila's presence without having to bother to ask anyone else. But what about other visitors? What reason could be found to explain their presence, other than that they had come to keep an eye on Valerie? Why would she *want* them to be there and what would they be doing?

Michael had recently reported that when Valerie was watching TV she would keep saying, 'I've seen it before.' Penny enquired as to whether Valerie said that sort of thing all the time, or just sometimes. Did she, for instance, make those sort of remarks in relation to racing or animal programmes? Michael said, 'definitely not'. Penny pointed out that Valerie had developed her own way of saying to him either that what she was watching did not make sense to her (unfamiliar) or that it did not interest her (boring). Penny suggested that more racing and animal programmes should be built into her daily diet, and that Michael should introduce other TV watching companions for Valerie so that they could take it in turns. It was so important that the benign repetition on which Valerie relied did not become tedious for everyone else.

This prompted Michael to sort out a video of the famous occasion a long, long time ago, when Valerie's favourite horse, Bounding Bandit, had won The Cup. He discovered that Valerie was happy to have it on, again and again. She never seemed to tire of it. She was often making connections with it by what seemed to Michael quite obscure conversational routes, when something quite different was being discussed. Penny was thrilled at this news, and urged Michael to get on the case and study what Valerie was saying. It emerged that almost anything could be connected in some way with the subject of the video: a mug of coffee . . . mug . . . cup . . . The Cup. Look at the time . . . nearly time for the off . . . I wonder if the race has started . . . The Cup. From that bit of SPOTting it soon emerged that all anyone had to do to explain themselves, assuming Valerie enquired what they were up to, was to murmur that they would love to see the video of The Cup some time. Valerie had no more questions, they were all answered in a single phrase – one she used all the time herself. Everyone became a member of the same club, the 'let's watch the video of The Cup' club, just like that. Which just left the question of what Valerie's bottom line might be.

THE BOTTOM LINE – ALTRUISTIC TRIGGER

When Penny first explained the whole notion of the bottom line to Michael, he (and to some extent she too) thought that 'Michael will really worry' would be the best response if Valerie should ever flatly refuse to do something and be at risk. When Sheila heard about this latest item to be ticked off on the Profile Checklist, however, she entirely disagreed. She suggested to Penny that however devoted Mrs T was to The Captain, the truth of the matter was that Mrs T cared about her horses more than anything else in this world, including The Captain. She painted a graphic picture of Valerie's 'strong will as a woman' and how she 'always has things done her way or no way'. In Sheila's view, no human being would have a hope of standing in Mrs T's way if Mrs T had decided on a particular course.

Penny wondered how Michael would take to being rather firmly sidelined in this way. Could he sign up to it? She knew that her father Sam had never succeeded in swallowing his pride in such a way. Sam always assumed that if he really put his foot down about something that he saw as common sense, his wife would automatically fall into line. Then Penny remembered the episode at Christmas when she had bowed to Sam's better judgement and allowed common sense to prevail. She would never do that now; she would have the necessary carer courage to explain how his own needs should come second to those of his wife. Now, with Michael, she would take a deep breath, find the best, most tactful way of explaining how – to Valerie – horses were more important than people, and pray that his self-esteem could take the blow. It was to Sheila that she turned for help. She went about it in her own way and was soon back on the phone with the good news, 'The Captain agrees!'

Penny greatly admired Michael's strength of character, a quality she had loved about her father in so many ways, and for the umpteenth time thought how much better Sam would have been able to manage Dorothy's dementia if SPECAL had been around when he needed it. She turned her thoughts back to Michael and Valerie: the main structure of the Care Profile was in place and she must turn the spotlight on support for the main carer. Where was Michael in all this?

THE CARER'S NEW PROJECT

In fact, Michael was doing really well. He had got the idea of what SPOTting was all about and was finding acceptable answers to many of the questions that Valerie asked. For example, Valerie had a friend called Jane whose husband had died. Valerie never failed to ask 'How is he?' every single time Jane dropped by. Several ways of replying were tried out and none seemed quite the business; in the meantime, Valerie kept on asking the question. She would bring the subject up in the evenings when Jane wasn't there and Michael didn't know which way to turn. Then he tried 'He's fine, he's very happy.' Valerie never asked the question again. 'SPECAL seems to work!' he said to Penny in a tone of voice that suggested to her that he was half-baffled, half-thrilled, and really not sure which. But one thing was for sure, things were gradually getting better up in Yorkshire.

Measuring success was clearly important to Michael, particularly as he was inclined to look on the gloomy side. When asked how he might spot his own success, he usually responded with some sort of version of 'I really don't know', said in a somewhat depressed voice. Penny persevered, and one day he volunteered that Valerie did now at times give him 'luscious kisses'. That seemed as good as anything Penny had found on any of the more conventional scales used to measure carer well-being.

Gradually, little by little, Michael was finding it possible to get away from Valerie's company without causing her distress and without feeling too much guilt himself. Penny asked him to choose his Carer's New Project: something entirely new and fascinating to him, an activity that he had never thought he would get round to in his life. Michael produced three possibilities and soon plumped for digital photography. Then he found himself having to identify exactly how he was going to take this forward. He wasn't allowed to rest until he could say who he was going to approach for help, and how. He decided on asking a neighbour to find a tutor and agreed that because it was another item on the Profile Checklist, he must get on with it. He also acknowledged that he could now get out of the house without upsetting Valerie and her wanting to come too, so there was little excuse. Importantly, he was now able to return to Valerie, having been away for a while, without being accused of all sorts of ghastly things, ending up in a disastrous argument as to where he had been and why he had not told her anything about it.

Although feeling more emotionally robust, Michael still found SPECAL counter-intuitive and difficult. He wrote to Penny that the recording of questions was hard – that when Valerie asked him something, because he couldn't record it straight away he forgot both the question and the answer he tried to give. He was still worrying about Valerie's role with the horses but finding that the idea of agreeing with her was hugely successful. He recorded:

> 'Valerie had a bad go about the horses the other day. She suddenly announced that she was going to have them all home and train them herself, which of course she could not do. I just said okay and left it at that. She did soon forget it. She then said she needed the *Racing Post* to do all the entries, which of course she does not do, and the trainers have her authority to act and they do the entries. I replied that I agreed and she did stop.'

NURSING HOME FOR THE FUTURE

Penny wanted to know which nursing home had been chosen by the family for the future, and the name of the manager there. Michael was still very reluctant to consider this subject at all, but eventually he fell into line. He set off on his search, and decided on Happylands, a home only a few miles away with a delightful manager, an Irish nurse trained in mental health by the name of Tommy. Tommy and Penny chatted on the phone, exchanged brochures, and agreed the basic principles of a transitional plan for Valerie, should this ever become desirable (or suddenly necessary) at some future point.

Once Michael had settled the nursing home question he seemed to be more confident about the future and started to ask when Valerie would go there. Penny explained that the aim for the moment was to get 'a day in the life of Valerie' established at home. Only when her 24-hour routine was up and running on a daily basis, and thoroughly green, would they think about moving her. In the meantime they must press on, because there could be a crisis at any time and the wraparound care was far from complete.

She told Michael how much his skills had developed, but he was not convinced and constantly chastised himself for not doing better. Penny was adamant. He was certainly not failing Valerie, in fact he was doing spectacularly well. 'On, on,' Penny repeatedly said. 'Oh all right!' now came the reply, 'What on earth comes next?' What came next was to identify the Tipping Point, which Penny privately thought was closer than anyone imagined, because Sheila was coming under a good deal of strain and could clearly not go on for ever in her ever more demanding role. Michael needed to get away on holiday from time to time and unless Valerie could remain at home while he was away, she would be far better making a single move into care.

Alas, Michael was still insisting on Valerie's daily routine being interrupted in some way and each occasion proved fairly disastrous. There was a trip to Deauville to see her horse running, an occasion which for Valerie became a re-run of The Cup victory. Her horse came in second, but when it came to the presentation of the winner's trophy she swept onto the podium and accepted it graciously, brushing the true winner out of the way. It was a totally disastrous occasion that took a lot of sorting out.

Then there were trips to Gozo where Michael and Valerie had spent holidays for many years. Penny kept transmitting the message, 'Do not go to Gozo' but Michael understandably wanted to keep returning and to have Valerie by his side.

There were problems packing. Valerie's case contained mountains of clothes including a woollen plus-four suit for shooting, several huge anoraks and masses of thick sweaters, along with 12 pairs of shoes. Problems at the airport were numerous as Valerie's hand luggage was closely inspected. Once they arrived, Valerie unpacked all her clothes, ironed them and replaced them in her suitcase ready to depart later that day. She repeatedly suggested to Michael that they go to Peter's house, and whenever a car passed them she would ask, 'Is that Peter?' On their return journey, Michael left the passports behind, so they missed the plane and Valerie was completely thrown. As soon as they arrived home she was convinced she was still in Gozo, and climbed all over Michael trying to get out of bed, as she had been sleeping on the other side in Gozo and couldn't make the switch back.

On one of their trips to Gozo they took Sheila, and her report of the fortnight took the hair off Penny's head. Clearly the Tipping

Point had been reached and passed, but before she could have any detailed discussion with Michael, Valerie managed to resolve the issue on her own. Back in Yorkshire, she had a most dramatic fall.

THE TIPPING POINT – A CRISIS

In the middle of the night in early December 2007 Michael woke up to hear Valerie shouting. It took him a bit of time to work out what was happening. When he called out 'Where are you?' she replied, 'Down here, in bed.' He asked her which room she was in and she replied, 'Don't be stupid!' Michael found her eventually, lying on her side having fallen downstairs and taken a picture off the wall as she flew down. She was transferred by ambulance to hospital, where she explained to the staff on arrival that she had been kicked by a horse. She was put in plaster from her toes to her hip and remained in hospital for a further week. With good reason was Michael terrified of how she would react to hospital. However, after a great deal of input from Sheila, using the various Themes and Explanations, the situation proved entirely manageable. Penny advocated taking Sheila over each day, so that she could be around to monitor what was going on. Michael also went over, and they took it in turns to sit with Valerie, boxing and coxing with their Explanations that worked as well in the ward as they had done at home.

Michael put the senior ward nurse in touch with Penny. She was extremely busy but most helpful, and together they quickly talked through the idea of the Themes and Explanations. Michael rang Tommy at Happylands, who turned up trumps with a bed almost immediately. Valerie was soon discharged straight from the hospital to Happylands, travelling calmly in a form of hospital transport which seemed to Valerie remarkably like a horsebox. The day of the move was planned like an army exercise, and mini-transitions between the ward and other parts of the hospital were rehearsed for several days beforehand. Sheila used to set off on expeditions with Valerie in a wheelchair to have coffee in the hospital canteen. Their conversation topics proved their worth when the day of the full transition arrived.

Before the move Michael and Sheila took a lot of Valerie's furniture and favourite possessions over to Happylands. They rang Penny to tell her how pleased they were to have got rid of all the nursing home furniture and made her room look so like the sitting room at home. Penny immediately counselled moving all Valerie's furniture out again and restoring a more institutional look. She explained that 18 years of experience of moving people with dementia into care had taught her that if you want to present something as a temporary hotel, it is not sensible to make it look like home: it will only confuse the person and make them wonder what is going on. Fortunately the owner had a good, Irish sense of humour and saw the funny side of the 'now you see it, now you don't' approach, and a place was found in Happylands to store all Valerie's furniture until after the move. This reassured Michael, because, as Penny pointed out, if Valerie did ask for any particular item, he only had to go down the corridor rather than transport it from home. She suggested that if Valerie hadn't asked for anything after, say, a couple of weeks, he could move it all back to his own home then.

A few very important items from Valerie's favourite possessions were left in the room. Two much-loved soft toys were waiting on her bed and her dressing gown was hung within sight, on the back of the door. There was a disc player set on repeat with a favourite selection of Ray Charles tunes, which were playing in the background when she first walked into the room. Everything else in the room, apart from some favourite flowers, belonged to the nursing home. The scene suggested a place in which to temporarily convalesce – 'a SPECAL hotel' as everyone called it – with only a very few carefully chosen props.

When Valerie arrived, Michael and Sheila were already in the home and remained out of sight, shadowing carefully. When Valerie first met the manager she picked up his Irish accent and before he could say much more than 'How nice to see you' she was in full flow, 'I know where you come from! You ought to come in as a sharer of the foal we are planning and we could race it as a syndicate!' The manager had studied the full transitional care plan including Valerie's Passport and understood how to respond. He thanked Valerie profusely, adding that he would give it some thought; although it would be a lot of money, it sounded a very good idea.

When Valerie was settled in to the room, Sheila wandered in as if she had been staying in the next door one. 'Gosh, you are lucky! This looks like a four-star hotel!' Valerie agreed and said she just hoped she could keep the room, which Sheila assured her she could. Within days, Valerie was talking of a party she was organising, explaining to the care assistants that they should come in black dresses and asking Sheila to do the cooking. At the end of a week, Sheila went in as usual to see Valerie and found her sitting in the corridor. She said, 'It's so lovely here. I really love it and I have got such a delightful room. You must come and see it.'

A few more days went by and Michael became concerned that Valerie might want to come home when her plaster was taken off. Penny suggested choosing his moment carefully and talking about convalescence, and if that went well, to recycle the conversation. Soon after that Michael reported that he had found Valerie sitting in a particular spot in the passage, where she could see the garden and where there was always somebody passing. She seemed very pleased to see him and 'we had a lovely smile and snuggle' and for the next half hour Valerie never mentioned anything at all about home.

On another occasion she saw two wheelchairs and asked Michael to decide which was best, as she would need one at home. She watched while Michael made a careful selection and then asked him to make sure that they book it. A care assistant passed by at that point and Valerie asked if she could take the red wheelchair home with her. 'Of course' said the care assistant, 'You can have whichever one you want.' Michael said to Valerie, 'They all seem to like you and that is why they are so helpful.' Valerie smiled with pleasure and said, 'I will miss them when I go home.'

Valerie was often sure she and Michael were on holiday as they sat together and that they were flying home the next day. She kept saying, 'I must do my packing.' One day she said, quite philosophically, 'I don't think this has been one of our better holidays. It has been rather boring.' This prompted Penny to suggest making sure that the *Racing Post* was always around the place and that the music player was on.

Many of Michael's diary entries were by now including success stories based on repetition. Phrases like 'you are marvellous' and 'you're so clever' came almost naturally to him these days. On several occasions he said to Valerie that he felt they were so lucky to have such a nice rehabilitation home and each time Valerie replied with a smile, 'Yes, I know.' Soon Michael was reporting that she was 'definitely on green the whole time'.

One day he felt sure she thought she was back in Gozo. She asked him what the weather forecast was, so he read it out of the paper and was promptly told that she did not want to hear 'the

English one'. She then turned to a man sitting on the other side of her and asked him whether he had been swimming. He looked a bit startled and said a very Yorkshire 'Nooo!' Valerie turned to Michael and repeated the same question. Michael replied, 'You know me. It is far too cold.' Michael was generally thrilled with how well everything had gone, while Penny warned that problems were bound to arise. She stressed that anything that did not go well should be monitored carefully: it would only be a matter of amber but it would need rapidly addressing to avoid it developing into a traumatic red.

Sure enough, trouble came a week later. Valerie had been walking about, putting weight on her leg and the staff kept trying to stop her. Valerie became aggressive and pushed them away. If the staff removed her Zimmer frame to discourage her from walking, she would merely set off to another resident's room in search of a replacement. When she found what she was looking for, she would try and remove it, often finding herself with an irate resident hanging on to the other end. Tommy explained to Michael that he could not have this sort of thing going on at Happylands and that he would like Valerie to be referred for a psychiatric review. Michael feared that tranquillisers would be prescribed and asked him if he would talk things over with Penny before he did anything else.

Penny prepared a risk management strategy form, based on a model from the Burford Hospital days, when all risk for dementia patients was managed by addressing the emotional factors of any issue first. The risk was identified as Valerie feeling disempowered if she were to be restrained by other people when she chose to move around the home without assistance. The strategy focused on staff ensuring that Valerie had her own Zimmer close at hand and offered to her if she wished to move about. She was then to be shadowed and any opportunity taken to offer a therapeutic pause in her travels. If she then chose to sit down, she should find herself within easy reach of a book about horses or flowers, or a copy of the *Racing Post*. If Valerie were to head for anyone else's Zimmer, she should be offered her own *before* the other Zimmer was taken away from her.

Tommy held a staff meeting and the risk management strategy was introduced. It worked wonders and soon Valerie was walking less, sitting more, and accepting help when it was offered. There were no more unseemly Zimmer frame fights.

Over the next few weeks several other incidents arose, and Tommy asked Penny to design further strategies in each case. These were all implemented with success. By now everyone was getting the measure of the approach, and the next step was to encourage Michael to visit less frequently. He took his duties very seriously and indeed loved his visits, but it was time for him to pick up on his own life as well. The farm and the horses needed him too. As he began, reluctantly at first, to visit less, he discovered that it made no difference whatsoever to Valerie whether he came every day or only once a week. He was always met with the same smile, just as if he had always been there.

Only recently Michael wrote to Penny with the following quotation of an exchange he had with Valerie:

VALERIE: I do love you. Please don't leave me.

MICHAEL: And I love you, and would not dream of leaving you.

VALERIE: Oh, that's good because I don't know what I would do without you.

MICHAEL: Well, you won't have to find out because I certainly could not do without you.

Postscript: SPECALSENSE Rules?

It is to be hoped that you have obtained from this book all the information that you need to provide SPECALCARE. Please do not hesitate to seek further advice and support by contacting SPECAL. If you look on the website www.specal.co.uk you will find details of how to make contact with expert advisers. For those who do not have access to the Internet, get someone you know who does to obtain the details. You may also find useful information at www.oliver-james-books.com.

At the time of writing, SPECAL has ambitious plans for making Penny Garner's work more widely known and these may be of interest to you.

SPECAL training around the country

Plans are afoot to train sufficient numbers of practitioners to provide face-to-face help to carers and professionals who want to attend workshops in the SPECAL method.

Training for nursing home staff

SPECAL hopes to reach a point where all nursing homes have at least one member of staff who has been trained to enable a SPECAL-informed transition of new clients when they first arrive at a nursing home.

Training for allied professions

SPECAL is contributing to government plans for provision for dementia. The goal is to ensure that all professionals who come into contact with clients with dementia are aware of the basic precepts of SPECALCARE.

Centre of Excellence at Burford

Since the publication of the hardback edition of this book in August 2008, several hundred professionals and family members have attended presentations and workshops at our Centre of Excellence at the Old Hospital at Burford. A number of professionals have also observed the work of Burford Practitioners interacting with clients. SPECAL is currently using only one third of the hospital premises, and is working on plans to return 24/7 services to the site at the earliest opportunity. This will increase the scope for observational sessions and offer the possibility of specialised placement for staff in training.

On a wider scale, there has been a gratifying amount of interest in SPECAL from political parties and we are hopeful that the approach will eventually become a key element in training and provision of care for all people with dementia in Britain.

Whatever comes of these plans, it is my earnest hope that carers everywhere will soon be aware that dementia does not need to be the gruesome nightmare that, at present, it all too often constitutes. Once you understand the disability using the tools developed by Penny, truly, you too can make a present of the client's past. I wish you the very best of luck in your invaluable and all too often unacknowledged efforts to do so.

Frequently Asked Questions

Q: If the SPECAL method is as effective as you claim, how come it has not been adopted wholesale by the Health and Social Services or the dementia charities, and how come I had never heard of it until I encountered this book?

A: Although Penny has been teaching her method to professionals from all over the world for several years, the vast majority of her clinical activity with carers and clients has been restricted to the Burford area. Her charity has very limited funds and its capacity to influence national provision has been restricted up until now.

Q: We are planning to go on our annual holiday in Cornwall shortly. I am worried that my husband will be even more confused than he was last year, but am reluctant to call it a day and break with tradition. What should I do?

A: Everything we do in life carries an element of risk, and in this case you need to weigh up the plusses and minuses of yet another Cornish holiday. Penny's mantra here would be 'grateful not greedy', and suggest that the Tipping Point in terms of yet more Cornish holidays has clearly been reached. Why not use the topic of Cornwall as a ping-pong ball, and identify the principal pleasures that a lifetime of Cornish holidays has already placed in the album? This is armchair travel of the most rewarding kind. You could then move on to find an acceptable explanation for why you might perhaps postpone the trip this year, on the 'what-if' basis, but do remember that you may never have to offer the explanation if the client doesn't ask. This is a case where you may well be able to use dementia as a positive resource, talking about, rather than going to, Cornwall this year.

Q: What are the main differences between the younger person with dementia and a person who develops dementia in much later life?

A: An important difference, from the SPECAL perspective, is that the younger person has comparatively fewer photographs in their album, and may have areas of unfulfilled ambition. They may have quite young children, whereas the older person may already have grandchildren. They may have a career still in front of them, whereas the older person may have already retired. The younger person may have a whole stack of places in the world they still wish to visit, whereas the older person may be beginning to feel that the place they like best is home. The idea of being grateful, not greedy, is far easier applied to the older person, and the notion of new being beautiful may be far more motivating to the younger person than someone of more advanced years. In a nutshell, the contrast between who the person was, shortly before the dementia impacted, and who they are now that they have been diagnosed, is far less for the older person. It may be important to 'buy time' and promote new activities for the younger person with dementia, whereas it may be more important to draw on what is already there in the album for the older person. For this reason, services for the younger person may have a different focus, in some important respects, from those aimed specifically at the older person.

Another difference is one of statistics. There are at least 20 times more older people than younger people diagnosed with dementia. Yet another is the rate at which the condition is liable to involve medical complications which would not have arisen without the arrival of dementia on the scene.

Q: My mother, who cares for my father with dementia, has inoperable cancer and has only a short time to live. Surely it is more important to ensure that my mother's last few months are peaceful, and we should prioritise her care needs over those of my father?

A: SPECAL is quite clear about the need to sort out your father's needs first, in order to ensure that your mother can have a peaceful end to her own life. The peace of mind which comes from knowing that the person with dementia is okay, which can be rapidly achieved, will bring untold benefit to your mother in her last few months. We know that where dementia is present, it invariably pays to make this the immediate, primary focus. This course of action will ensure that everyone has peace of mind. The reverse simply doesn't work.

Q: Can anyone provide SPECALCARE?

A: Yes, if you have an open mind.

Q: My husband constantly denies that he has a problem. Does this mean it isn't worth my following the method?

A: No. By following the SPECAL principles, life will be easier for both of you.

Q: How can I involve my wife in what I am doing with the book?
A: Follow the SPECALSENSE involved in the book.

Q: Is it ever too late for SPECALCARE?
A: No, but the earlier you start the easier it will make your lives.

Q: Is it ever too early for SPECALCARE?
A: No, because the sooner you understand how to manage the situation, the easier it will be for the client, carer and others involved.

Q: When you say to start SPECALCARE early, how early is early?
A: As soon as diagnosis is made. You need to develop the Profile and start using it so that you can gradually increase it to keep pace with the degree of blanking as time goes by.

Q: Why does the carer have to do something new, rather than go back to an interest that they have loved in the past and had to give up?
A: Because it has to be a challenge and a new interest to allow the carer to really focus on a New Project that will fully take them away from their daily caring routine for gradually increasing periods.

Q: Surely there's no point in choosing a nursing home very far ahead?

A: It takes time to choose the most appropriate place and to build a relationship, book a provisional place and, not least, to determine the financial implications. You do not know how quickly the client's condition may deteriorate.

Q: My husband has just been diagnosed at the age of 51. Surely he will feel demeaned if I tell him that he should leave everything to me from now on?

A: SPECALSENSE is not a recipe for demeaning your husband, but rather for ensuring that his lifestyle from now on is as close as possible to the one he would have led without dementia. You are asking him to trust you to act on his behalf in terms of anything new (and therefore comparatively complex) from now on, so that you can both continue to enjoy life with confidence.

Q: Why doesn't everyone use SPECAL if it is as great as it is purported to be?

A: Because it is not well known. It has a single research base in the Burford, Oxfordshire area and due to limited funds and resources, the knowledge has not yet been widely disseminated through trained trainers.

Q: My mother has dementia and my father is caring for her. I know that my mother expects my father to make the decisions, but he has asked me to help out. I am wondering whether I should explain this to my mother, so that I can be sure she is happy for me to be helping in this way?

A: SPECALSENSE points the way to making things as simple as possible, without losing sight of the ethical issues involved. Provided your mother has made it clear that your father is the person she most trusts – in other words, that he is her most significant other – then clearly he must be able to delegate tasks in order to fulfil his promise to your mother that he will look after her best interests. No one person can do everything, and the cascade of consent from the client to the most significant other makes profound SPECALSENSE. Given that it is imperative to avoid questions to the client as soon as possible after diagnosis, it becomes obvious that the primary consent from client to most significant other must lead to, but not exclude, responsible delegation.

Q: My partner denies that there is anything wrong whatsoever. Should I agree?

A: Yes. As a first step, never contradict. However you can find ways of saying that it is as well for you both to remain on the look-out for any signs of unusual memory loss, simply because there is so much that can be done to avoid it becoming a real problem, provided it is picked up at an early stage. You can also say that you are watching your own memory carefully, and reading a bit about the subject, just so you know what to look out for.

Q: What is SPECAL's view of drugs?

A: The Royal College of Nursing found that SPECAL clients take fewer drugs and experience less distress. The application of a SPECAL Profile, and associated risk management strategies, will ensure that medication is kept at the lowest possible level at all times.

SPECAL Contact Details

The SPECAL Centre
Sheep Street
Burford
OX18 4LS

Email: help@specal.co.uk
Website: www.specal.co.uk

Acknowledgements

First and foremost, I must acknowledge Penny Garner, who devised the method described in this book. It is an extraordinary achievement to have invented it. She has been unstinting in her time in conveying it to me and endlessly long-suffering in explaining its finer points when I have failed to grasp them. Thank you Penny. I cannot stress strongly enough the degree to which I have been at best a Boswell to her Johnson. Both the theory and the practice described in these pages are wholly hers.

I also want to pay tribute to the significant contribution made to SPECAL by Penny's nuclear family, whom she describes as having stoically survived periods of considerable neglect over many years: her loyal husband William Garner, whose generosity and forbearance has been crucial, and her daughters Clare, Anna-Louise and Emma, for their cheerful acceptance of SPECAL as an adopted sibling. Each family member has brought their own talents to bear in nurturing SPECAL since its beginning in the late eighties.

I would particularly like to thank my wife Clare for suggesting the idea of writing a book about Penny's work and for supporting me so considerately throughout, however demanding the schedule and however erratic my state of mind.

As always, thanks to Jemima Biddulph for editing this book and for pointing out when it was going in the wrong direction.

At Vermilion, particular thanks to Fiona MacIntyre for seeing the potential in this book. Thanks to Anna Hervé for her help. Thanks to Julia Kellaway for her in-house editing work. Thanks also to Caroline Brown and Sarah Bennie in the publicity department.

At my agent's, Aitken Alexander, Gillon served his usual rock-solid role and Clare Alexander helped us to get everything on the road in a most effective manner.

Finally, my thanks to the many people who have given of their time and other resources to enable SPECAL to flourish throughout its remarkable history, and to those who are supporting it today in so many different ways.

Index

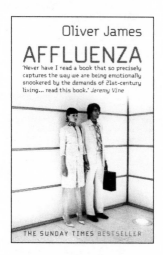

The Selfish Capitalist

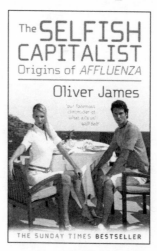

In the bestselling *Affluenza*, Oliver James introduced us to a modern-day virus sweeping through the world. Now *The Selfish Capitalist* provides more detailed substantiation for the claims made in *Affluenza*. It looks deeper into the origins of the virus and outlines the political, economic and social climate in which it has grown as James provides a wealth of evidence to show that we have become more miserable and distressed since the seventies.

A rallying cry to the government to reduce our levels of distress by adopting a form of unselfish capitalism, this hard-hitting and thought-provoking work tells us why our personal well-being must take precedence over the wealth of a tiny minority if we are to cure ourselves of this epidemic.

£8.99   9780091924164

Order this title direct from www.oliver-james-books.com